HEAL YOUR FROZEN SHOULDER

An At-Home Rehab Program to End Pain and Regain Range of Motion

Dr. Karl Knopf

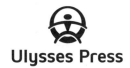

Ulysses Press

Published in the United States by:
Ulysses Press
P.O. Box 3440
Berkeley, CA 94703
www.ulyssespress.com

ISBN: 978-1-61243-643-2
Library of Congress Control Number: 2016950674

Printed in the United States by Kingery Printing Company
10 9 8 7 6 5 4 3

Acquisitions editor: Casie Vogel
Managing editor: Claire Chun
Editor: Lily Chou
Proofreader: Renee Rutledge
Indexer: Sayre Van Young
Front cover/interior design: what!design @ whatweb.com
Layout: Jake Flaherty
Cover artwork: © Rapt Productions except woman with blue exercise band © lightwavemedia/shutterstock.com
Interior artwork: © Rapt Productions except pages 8, 10 © Sebastian Kaulitzki/shutterstock.com
Models: Evan Clontz, Kym Sterner, Chris Wells, Chris Knopf

Distributed by Publishers Group West

CONTENTS

Part 3: MAINTENANCE, STRENGTHENING & CONDITIONING EXERCISES — 95

Chapter 6: POST-INJURY: KEEPING YOUR SHOULDER STRONG AND HEALTHY 95

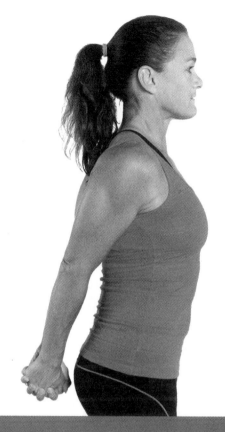

Part 1

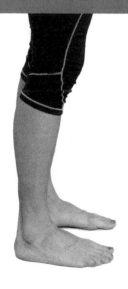

GETTING STARTED

INTRODUCTION

Frozen shoulder is a mysterious condition in which the connective tissues around the shoulder joint thicken and tighten, leading to loss of mobility. Basically, your shoulder "freezes" up. The technical definition of frozen shoulder is adhesive capsulitis, which is the medical term for stiffness and pain associated with limited range of movement in the shoulder. It most often occurs in just one shoulder but can occur in both.

Shoulder dysfunction is caused by many variables: falls, overuse, misuse, and even disuse after an injury. Injury to the soft tissue surrounding the shoulder joint may very well be prevented if you perform a gentle strengthening program of corrective exercises, but if you currently have a frozen shoulder you may already know this and now want to get better. The good news is that 90 percent of frozen shoulders can be rehabilitated. Patience and a regular schedule of gentle exercises are key.

The intent of this book is to offer you corrective exercises that you can do over a lifetime to prevent the condition from returning. The book will give a brief overview of shoulder anatomy, describe frozen shoulder dysfunction, and provide corrective and post-rehab exercises.

This book is not meant to be a replacement or a substitute for medical care or physical therapy. For the best chance of full recovery, all treatment plans should be designed with your individual characteristics in mind. With the supervision of a doctor and therapist, anyone can use this book to improve range of motion and strengthen the shoulder region. The information contained within this book has been gleaned from medical publications and therapy handbooks and represents the most current information about frozen shoulder. However, as with anything, as further clinical research is done, treatment plans may change.

WHO GETS SHOULDER ISSUES?

Statics show that, over a lifetime, more than 20 percent of the adult population has or will suffer from a shoulder joint dysfunction that affects daily activities. A shoulder dysfunction is no small problem; it can disable a person for a sustained period of time. The causes of shoulder problems are many and varied and can range from improper body mechanics, such as sitting incorrectly at the computer, or too many overhead movements. Who gets frozen shoulder issues?

- People who engage in repetitive overhead motions are more prone to shoulder pain and dysfunction.

- People who have prolonged immobilization of the joint due to pain or poor rehab.

- Women are more frequently affected than men.

- Those with a history of diabetes have a higher incidence than non-diabetics.

- Older people—incidence increases with age.

While age doesn't cause shoulder problems, it unfortunately brings changes in joint structures and soft tissues of the shoulder joint. As we age, the soft tissues surrounding the shoulder girdle undergo some structural changes that often lead to the weakening of the supporting ligaments, tendons, and muscles.

Some experts in the field suggest that, by 50 years of age, most people have some internal shoulder structural changes. Often, tendinitis can manifest itself as a tendon degenerates with age and misuse. If simple chronic shoulder issues aren't properly treated early, greater damage can occur—which is why early intervention and preventative maintenance are the key to complete shoulder health.

The occurrence of frozen shoulder is seen more frequently in people with a history of diabetes, or chronic inflammatory arthritis of the shoulder, or those who have had chest or breast surgery as well as a stroke. It's very common to see a person who experiences shoulder pain try to protect the joint by not moving it. Any long-term immobility of the shoulder joint can put people at risk of developing a frozen shoulder.

DO I HAVE A SHOULDER ISSUE?

The onset of a shoulder problem often manifests slowly over time and is neglected until it affects the person's range of motion or the pain is unbearable. Ironically, the natural response to stop using the shoulder when it hurts may actually contribute to a frozen shoulder.

Unfortunately, many people wait too long before going to the doctor about their shoulder problem, assuming it will just get better on its own. Research suggests that most people don't go to the doctor until they've lost some level of range of motion. The current belief is that proactive steps such as medical care and gentle movement are the keys to preventing frozen shoulder syndrome.

If you suspect that you have a shoulder issue, get a diagnosis ASAP. An early intervention can keep a small issue from becoming a big one. Make an appointment with your primary care doctor, who's usually the port of entry into the medical system. Your general doctor may then refer you to other health professionals.

Some signs that you may have a shoulder problem are:

- Difficulty moving a computer mouse around on the desk
- Pain when reaching upward, such as when putting groceries away on a high shelf
- Hearing a shoulder "pop" after throwing a ball for your dog or after serving an ace in tennis
- Discomfort when reaching into your back pocket to grab your wallet or when pulling up a back zipper on a dress

WHAT SHOULD I EXPECT WHEN VISITING THE DOCTOR?

When meeting with your health professional, explain to her all your functional limitations, such as difficulty or pain when:

- Putting on a coat
- Sleeping on your side

- Reaching behind you or to a high shelf

- Throwing a ball overhand

- Performing work duties

- Participating in recreational pursuits

Additionally, come prepared to share the type of work performed as well as your fitness routines, recreational pursuits, and any recent injuries. The more information you can provide will assist the health professional in developing a treatment plan. Don't be discouraged—sometimes in the case of a frozen shoulder the cause isn't known.

Expect that the doctor will take a detailed health history as well as complete a comprehensive physical exam, possibly moving your arm through different motions while comparing it to your non-involved side. The doctor may order some X-rays to be taken of the shoulder to assist in making a diagnosis. You may receive a referral to a physical therapist, who might perform a biomechanical evaluation to look for any postural deviations and functional limitations. All these evaluations will assist in making a correct diagnosis and developing a proper treatment plan, which might include medications, physical therapy, and a home-care program.

Chapter 1

SHOULDER ANATOMY

The shoulder, more accurately called the "shoulder girdle," is a remarkable joint. It can gently toss an egg back and forth, rock a baby to sleep, hurl a baseball at 90 mph, and generate a 100-mph serve in tennis. The shoulder is much more than a single joint. This complex joint is where bones come together and are surrounded and supported by soft tissue, which includes ligaments, tendons, and bursas. Most experts maintain that the shoulder joint consists of the following bones: the humerus, scapular, and clavicle. Some experts even include the rib cage, thoracic, and cervical aspects of the spine.

An engineering marvel, the shoulder joint's design allows for maximum flexibility and function in almost every conceivable direction. This mobility, however, is also why the shoulder girdle, a ball-and-socket joint, is so vulnerable to overuse and injuries, and one reason why it's the most difficult and complicated joint in the body to rehabilitate.

The current philosophy in health care today is "knowledge is power." To help you understand why certain treatment and exercise plans are beneficial to rehabilitating and preventing a frozen shoulder, here's a basic overview of the shoulder anatomy and its kinesiology. Understanding your condition will help you follow through with the steps needed to fully recover.

BONES & JOINTS

The shoulder joint consists of a large ball and smaller socket. The basic structure is similar to a sideway-lying golf tee with a tennis ball next to it, held in place with a series of bands called ligaments and tendons. Ligaments attach bone to bone while tendons attach muscle to bone. This anatomical design, unfortunately, doesn't provide a great deal of structural support. Generally, in the human body, extensive flexibility at a joint also means reduced stability. By comparison, the hip is also a ball-and-socket joint, but it's a deep ball and socket, which provides a great deal of structural support but not much mobility.

The normal shoulder joint function allows for:

- Flexion and extension

- Horizontal and lateral adduction and abduction

- Internal and external rotation

- Upward and downward scapular motion

The shoulder girdle is composed of four bones. The *clavicle* is commonly known as the collar bone. The *scapula* is also known as the shoulder blades, or wing/angel bones. The *acromion* is the part of the scapula that forms a bony roof above the rotator cuff, tendons, and bursa. The *sternum* is often referred to as the breast bone. The *humerus* is the upper bone of the arm.

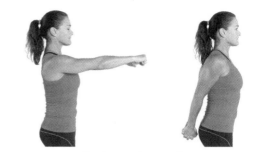

Flexion and extension

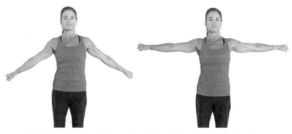

Horizontal and lateral adduction and abduction

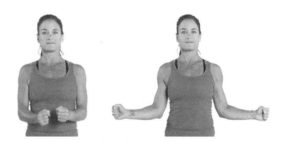

Internal and external rotation

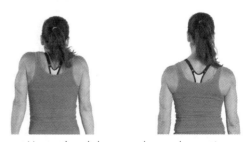

Upward and downward scapular motion

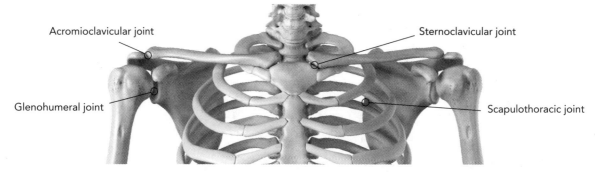

Acromioclavicular joint

Sternoclavicular joint

Glenohumeral joint

Scapulothoracic joint

Shoulder joints

Joints, where bones come together, are surrounded by soft tissue, which includes ligaments, tendons, and bursas.

There are several joints/articulations of the shoulder. The majority of the joint movement occurs in the glenohumeral joint; the other joints serve more as supporting structures.

Acromioclavicular (AC)—This joint is formed by the acromion and the clavicle. Mainly, it's active with shrugging movements.

Glenohumeral (GH)—The combination of the upper arm bone and the outside area of the scapula makes up this joint. This joint is responsible for most of the movements of the shoulder. Shoulder dislocation always refers to this joint.

Sternoclavicular (SC)—This joint is composed of the clavicle and the sternum. This joint primarily operates during shrugs, although part of its function is to stabilize the shoulder girdle.

Scapulothoracic (ST)—This isn't really a movable joint but serves as a base for muscles to be secured to.

Each of the four rotary cuff muscles (see Muscles on page 9) originates on the scapula and their tendons attach to the top of the humerus, helping to form the joint capsule.

THE SUPPORTING CAST

LIGAMENTS AND TENDONS

The shoulder joint's ligaments and tendons impart stability, but these bands can become lax through misuse and chronic overuse. Each type of fiber has a unique role to play and offers different abilities. Some shoulder experts call these elements the "passive system." All this complexity allows the shoulder joint to be one of the most mobile joints of the body. This mobility, however, is also why the shoulder joint is so vulnerable to overuse and injuries, and one reason why it's the most difficult and complicated joint in the body to rehabilitate.

Ligaments attach bone to bone while tendons attach muscle to bone. Ligaments are not just some simple set of guide wires; they twist and turn to provide stability along with providing neuromuscular feedback via the proprioceptive nervous system. Often with age these ligaments lose tensile strength, setting up a potential for injury. The ligaments of the shoulder region are the acromioclavicular ligament, also known as the AC joint ligament, and the coracoclavicular ligament.

THE JOINT CAPSULE

CARTILAGE

Cartilage is the gristle/pad between joints, providing cushion. The cartilage is designed to provide a smooth surface for joint bones to glide over. Often, with use, these once-smooth surfaces wear down. Once they break down, as seen in osteoarthritis, pain and inflammation occur.

BURSA

The sac surrounding the joint is called a bursa. A fluid-filled bursa is usually found between bones and tendons to help decrease friction during normal joint use. It provides lubrication to the joint. Many times, after frequent insults and impingements, the bursa becomes inflamed, causing pain that can lead to restricted movement.

MUSCLES

Before we move on to the muscles of the shoulder, remember that muscles can do two things: contract or relax. *Agonist muscles* are responsible for contraction movements, while *antagonist muscles* produce an action opposite of the agonist. In addition, *stabilizer muscles* anchor or support a bone so the agonist can have a firm base from which to operate (the rotator cuff muscles are a good example of a stabilizer muscle).

The major muscles of the shoulder region are sometimes broken down into either static stabilizers (SS) or dynamic stabilizers (DS) of the joint. The muscles below serve to influence the motions available at the shoulder joint.

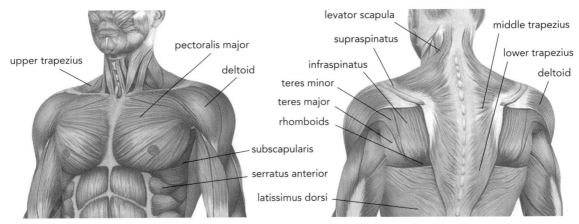

Shoulder muscles

Static stabilizers:

- Supraspinatus abducts the arm (i.e., moves the arm away from the body).

- Infraspinatus rotates the arm laterally.

- Teres minor rotates the arm laterally.

- Teres major adducts the arm (i.e., brings the arm in to the body).

- Subscapularis internally rotates the arm.

Dynamic stabilizers (prime movers):

- Latissimus dorsi extends and adducts the arm.

- Trapezius elevates and depresses the scapula.

- Pectoralis major and minor adduct the arm and pull the scapula downward.

- Coracobrachialis flexes and adducts the arm.

- Deltoid abducts and extends the arm.

- Levator scapula moves the neck laterally.

- Rhomboid major and minor stabilize the scapula.

- Serratus anterior stabilizes the scapula.

Other than trauma and repetitive chronic misuses, muscle imbalances, whether caused by work duties or recreational activities, are the prime culprit when it comes to shoulder injury. If one set of muscles gets too tight, the delicate balance of the space in the shoulder complex is upset, possibly throwing the alignment out of place. This is similar to the guide wires of a radio tower; if they're too tight, they can cause misalignment. These misalignments set the stage for injury. When the alignment of the joint is proper, ideal range of motion is expected.

Many times the cause of a shoulder problem can be traced back to misuse, overuse, disuse, or abuse of the shoulder joint and its supporting systems. Very often, postural deviations or muscle imbalances as a result of job duties or recreational activities can contribute to shoulder issues.

The muscles that are often implicated as being too tight and contributing to a shoulder imbalance are the:

- Trapezius (upper region)

- Levator scapula

- Sternocleidomastoid

- Internal rotators

- Pectoralis major and minor

- Latissimus dorsi

The muscles commonly found to be too weak are:

- Trapezius (middle and lower region)

- Rhomboids

- Serratus anterior

- External rotators

Perhaps if we followed Joseph Pilates' advice of strengthening what is weak and stretching what is tight, possibly some of our shoulder issues would've never occurred.

Chapter 2

FROZEN SHOULDER DYSFUNCTION

Shoulder problems can affect everyone, from office workers hunched over a computer and construction workers to homeowners who paint a bedroom wall and weekend athletes.

A frozen shoulder can be the result of inflammation, scarring, thickening, or shrinkage of the capsule that surrounds the normal shoulder capsule. Any injury to the shoulder region that leads to the formation of scar tissue of the shoulder capsule can contribute to a frozen shoulder. Commonly reported injuries that can lead to a frozen shoulder include tendinitis, bursitis, or a rotator cuff injury. Long-term immobility of the shoulder joint can also put people at risk to develop a frozen shoulder.

Frozen shoulder conditions are seen more often in people between the ages of 40 and 70 years, and more often in women (60 percent) versus men (40 percent). Frozen shoulder occurs more often in people with diabetes (15–20 percent) than those without diabetes (3–5 percent). Sometimes the etiology of the issues is idiopathic, meaning there's no known cause.

1. Injury to the shoulder region can cause trigger inflammation and scarring, as well as other structural changes to the joint capsule that surrounds the shoulder joint, contributing to a loss of mobility to the shoulder joint.

2. Both diabetes and osteoarthritis can contribute to frozen shoulder issues.

3. Often after breast cancer surgery and/or radiation, patients may have tight shoulder and chest muscles. This can contribute to decreased range of motion and develop into a frozen shoulder. This is why many physicians recommend that a post-surgery rehabilitation program be instituted.

4. Often, a long-term effect of a cerebral vascular accident (also known as a stroke or brain attack) can be frozen shoulder syndrome. This is why a proactive post-rehab program is critical to maintain functional range of motion.

5. Falling and trying to catch yourself with an outstretched arm can cause trauma to the shoulder region, contributing to a deficit in shoulder mobility.

SYMPTOMS

Your shoulder is designed to move freely in many directions. When pain limits your movement, you may likely decrease your range of motion. This reduction of motion can allow adhesions to develop and your shoulder appears to seize or "freeze" up, hence the name. As these adhesions develop, they can make movement more difficult and painful—leading to further reduction of motion and a frozen shoulder. This cycle of disuse sets up more pain and more immobility.

Here are some common symptoms:

- Pain in all directions

- Reduced range of motion

- Shoulder pain when lying on it

- Shoulder stiffness

The condition usually comes on insidiously, almost so slowly that people often dismiss it until they can't move the arm freely. In best-case situations, the shoulder can slowly improve over the course of a year or more, but in most cases, some intervention needs to occur.

There are four stages of frozen shoulder:

Stage 1: Inflammation. This stage can last 6 to 12 weeks.

Stage 2: Freezing. This stage, often associated with increased pain, can last up to six months.

Stage 3: Frozen. Improvement occurs slowly over four to six months, with pain decreasing but stiffness still lasting.

Stage 4: Thawing. This stage can last six months to two years before your shoulder returns to normal.

In most cases, full recovery eventually occurs with the use of NSAIDs, injections, and corrective exercise.

ASSESSMENT

Anyone with limited motion of the shoulder joint should seek the medical attention of a health care professional immediately. This is why early intervention with gentle passive and active exercises are generally recommended in the first place—to prevent the shoulder from freezing up.

During your assessment, your doctor will take a detailed health history and conduct a physical exam. Underlying diseases involving the shoulder can be diagnosed by blood testing, evaluating your range of motion, and pain of the involved joint. The diagnosis can be confirmed with an X-ray using a contrast dye that's injected into the shoulder joint. The tissues of the shoulder can also be evaluated with an MRI scan or by performing an arthroscopy, a minor surgical procedure where a scope is inserted into the joint through a small incision.

TREATMENT

The treatment of a frozen shoulder usually requires a combination of anti-inflammatory medications, cortisone injection(s) into the shoulder, and physical therapy. An exercise program developed by a physical therapist can help increase your range of motion. Without treatment, a frozen shoulder can become a permanent limitation. Diligent formal and home physical therapy is often the key to full restoration. Most cases of frozen shoulder can be improved with conservative care and time.

Massage therapy and manual therapy can be helpful. Physical therapy can take weeks to months for recovery, depending on the severity of the scarring of the tissues around the shoulder. It's very important for people with a frozen shoulder to avoid reinjuring the shoulder tissues during the rehabilitation period. Until fully recovered, it's critical to avoid:

- Sudden and jerking motions with the affected shoulder
- Heavy lifting with the affected shoulder
- Prolonged overhead activities
- Poor biomechanical maneuvers

Often, your doctor will suggest the following options to treat your frozen shoulder:

- Gentle shoulder stretches/range-of-motion exercises
- Anti-inflammatory medications
- Mild and moist heat
- Ice applications and ice massage
- Physical therapy or manual therapy and modalities
- Home mobility and conditioning program

If conservative care fails, additional medical treatments can include:

- Cortisone injections
- Surgical interventions and manipulations

Once released from formal therapy, a home health program should be initiated. Depending on the duration and severity of the frozen shoulder, full recovery is anticipated, yet in some cases, permanent loss of range of motion of the shoulder does occur. It's only with continued exercise of the shoulder that mobility and function is optimized. It's always recommended to get a comprehensive treatment plan from your health provider. (*Suggestion:* Take this book along to your next appointment and ask your health provider to design a program for you from the exercises displayed in this book.)

A frozen shoulder can take a year or more to get better. Good news: Most people will get better with time. Bad news: Most people get better with time.

The point of the above double message is that, given enough time, most shoulder issues resolve themselves. Unfortunately, some incidences of frozen shoulders can be resistant to conservative treatment, thus requiring other, more invasive treatments such as release of the scar tissue by a surgical procedure or manipulation of the scarred shoulder under anesthesia. This manipulation is performed to break up the scar tissue of the joint capsule and carries some risks that should be discussed with your health provider. It's very important for patients that undergo manipulation to partake in an active exercise program for the shoulder after the procedure.

PREVENTION

Can frozen shoulder be prevented? A proactive approach that includes proper body mechanics, a regular dose of gentle range-of-motion exercises, and a shoulder-conditioning program to develop agonist and anti-agonist muscles as well as stabilizers may prevent frozen shoulder from occurring. This may include strengthening lax muscles and improving flexibility of overly tight muscles. Unfortunately, sometimes it may not be possible to prevent frozen shoulder—as the saying goes, bad things happen to good people. But seeing the doctor at the early onset of even a simple limitation of mobility is wise: plus, following your doctor's advice can decrease the risk of developing a prolonged case of frozen shoulder.

OTHER CHRONIC CONDITIONS

While the focus of this book is on frozen shoulder, it's important to discuss other shoulder conditions that may contribute to a frozen shoulder. The following section provides an overview of many common shoulder dysfunctions such as arthritis, a fall to the shoulder region, tendinitis, or bursitis, as well repetitive motion issues and several more of the most common contributing factors. Sometimes the residual effects of a stroke can lead to frozen shoulder syndrome. It's always wise to consult your doctor for an accurate diagnosis of your shoulder.

While age is not the cause of frozen shoulder, it unfortunately does play a role in shoulder conditions. As we age, the soft tissues surrounding the shoulder girdle undergo some structural changes. Often, these structural changes lead to the weakening of the supporting ligaments, tendons, and muscles. Some experts in the field suggest that by 50 years of age, most people have some internal shoulder structural changes. Often, a simple tendinitis can degenerate into actual tearing of the tissues. If simple tendinitis is not properly treated, further episodes can lead to larger tears and greater damage—that's why early intervention and preventative maintenance are the key to complete shoulder health.

ARTHRITIS

Osteoarthritis of the shoulder is a degenerative condition in which the cartilage deteriorates, causing mild to moderate pain in the shoulder area as well as limited range of motion that contributes to the manifestation of a frozen shoulder syndrome. This is often the result of chronic wear and tear. However, it can be caused by disease, trauma, or infection. Arthritis of the shoulder is seen in the AC joint earlier than the GH joint because the AC joint degenerates more quickly. Arthritis's inflammation, pain, and restricted motion can be factors in the development of a frozen shoulder.

TENDINITIS AND BURSITIS

Tendinitis and bursitis are closely related and may occur alone or in combination. In *tendinitis* of the shoulder, the rotator cuff and/or biceps tendon become inflamed, usually as a result of being pinched by surrounding structures. The injury may vary from mild inflammation to involvement of most of the rotator cuff. When the rotator cuff tendon becomes inflamed and thickened, it may get trapped beneath the acromion. Squeezing of the rotator cuff is called *impingement syndrome*. Tendinitis and impingement syndrome are often accompanied by inflammation of the bursa sacs that are designed to protect the shoulder. An inflamed bursa is called *bursitis*. Inflammation, which is common with tendinitis and bursitis, can contribute to a frozen shoulder because often if something "hurts," the person favors or guards the area; thus, the lack of motion leads to the frozen shoulder.

SHOULDER IMPINGEMENT

Have you ever felt pinching when raising your arm? Do you have pain with movement or when lying on your side? Shoulder impingement is a somewhat common chronic condition.

Shoulder impingement can be caused by repetitive activity that requires the shoulder joint to do overhead motions day in and day out, such as tennis, doing home repairs, or even just sleeping on the same arm each night. Often this overuse condition causes pain and stiffness, and if a person does not seek proper medical care, they will guard the region, and over time, adhesions will develop, contributing to a frozen shoulder.

REPETITIVE MOTION INJURIES (RMI)

Anyone who uses the same arm over and over again for either work or recreation is at risk for repetitive motion injuries, also known as cumulative trauma disorder. These repetitive movements can aggravate your shoulder joint structures, such as the tendons, ligaments, bursa sac, or cartilage. If left unchecked, RMI can lead to inflammation and decreased range of motion.

Chapter 3

PREVENTING A FROZEN SHOULDER

We're all familiar with the saying "An ounce of prevention is worth a pound of cure." This concept is very relevant in preventing an injury and protecting your shoulder joint. We all understand that preventing a problem is a wise idea. We understand that concept when it comes to our automobile, whether it's a regular oil change or tune-ups. Preventive maintenance can prevent a breakdown or an expensive repair. Unfortunately, when it comes to our bodies, we neglect that basic advice.

The best defense against a frozen shoulder and other shoulder problems is becoming proactive. If you wish to avoid the drudgery of rehabilitation, consider performing pre-habilitation exercises as part of your daily routine. This type of approach involves a comprehensive general conditioning program with specific stretching and strengthening exercises aimed at toning the stabilizing structures as well as maintaining normal range of motion. Joseph Pilates (the father of Pilates exercises) said it best: "Stretch what is tight, and strengthen what is lax." While strength training is a good thing, too much can cause tightness and possible injury. While stretching is a good thing, too much can lead to a lax joint and possible injury.

TIPS FOR A HEALTHY SHOULDER

Be proactive about your shoulder. Early intervention of a problem keeps small problems small; what you do today determines your shoulder health tomorrow. Be aware of when to rest and recover so that you don't overwork your shoulder. Consider incorporating heat and ice into your workout. Most doctors suggest moist heat to loosen up a joint, followed by active warm-up to foster range of motion, followed by ice after your activity. You know how your shoulder feels—listen to it and heed what it says! Don't push through pain.

Train smart. It's crucial to have a well-designed fitness and sports program that balances volume and intensity of training. The program should include exercises that train the small supporting muscles and avoid any high-risk shoulder exercises (see Dangerous Dozen on page 27). Cross-training is important as it helps to prevent overuse syndrome.

Do it right. Learn proper biomechanics for work and play. Pay close attention to your head and upper back position during all activities. Poor form = poor function. Executing movements properly can prevent issues. Part of doing any exercise right is knowing your safe range of motion, which is different for each individual. One person's range may be another person's strain. It's a good idea to get your movement patterns evaluated by a trainer. Lastly, be mindful of your movements—avoid uncontrolled movements.

POSTURE'S ROLE IN PREVENTION

The interplay between poor posture and shoulder problems is beginning to be better understood. Most people know that poor posture can lead to back pain, but posture also plays an important role in shoulder health.

For instance, the rounded-shoulder, forward-head posture (think turtle) is often seen in people who swim a lot using the crawl/freestyle stroke without strengthening the opposing muscle group and stretching the chest muscles. Viewed from the front, such a swimmer has a fantastic physique but when viewed from the side, the swimmer displays a posture of a hunched-over old man.

This decreased flexibility of the chest and shoulder can set the stage for shoulder problems. Experts now understand that if one body part is misaligned, overused, or hurt, it can affect the mechanics elsewhere along the kinetic chain.

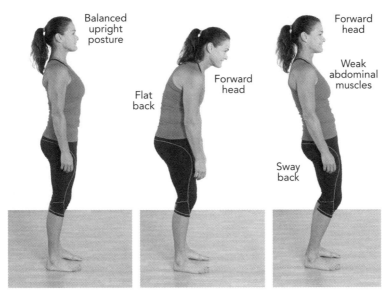

Balanced upright posture

Flat back

Forward head

Forward head

Weak abdominal muscles

Sway back

Proper posture (left) and poor posture (center, right)

Look at the image of good posture. Notice that the ear, shoulder, hip, and ankle are all on the same vertical line. Any deviation from this alignment can lead to a multitude of issues, from neck and shoulder problems to lower-back pain. Of course, plenty of things, like working a desk job, sitting in a cramped airplane seat, and fixing a car will challenge your ability to maintain good posture. That's why you should assess your posture several times a day.

The easiest way to do this is to stand with your back against a wall with your heels no more than 6 inches from the wall. Place your bottom to the wall and then attempt to place your upper back and the base of your head to the wall, keeping your chin down. If you have very compromised posture, start with just placing your bottom against the wall; as you improve, take your time trying to get your upper back against the wall before finally attempting to get your head to the wall. Some older people with severely compromised posture never get their head to the wall, so start today before it's too late. Practicing proper posture will reduce issues in all parts of the body, from head to toe.

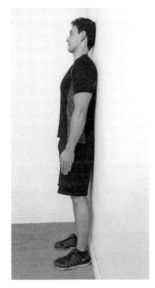

Assessing your posture

KNOW YOUR ZONES

Too often, people hurt their shoulder because they're not paying attention to how they're using it. If you've had a shoulder injury before, you should be particularly careful. One movement that commonly triggers a shoulder problem is simply overreaching, or surpassing your safe range of motion. If you imagine your range of motion as green, yellow, and red zones, staying mindful of this concept may prevent many shoulder issues.

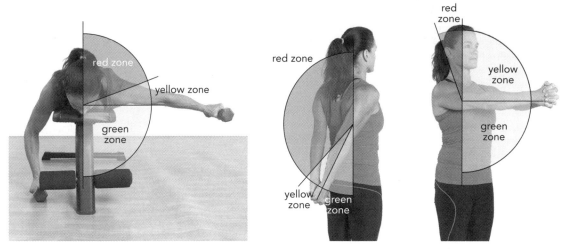

Range-of-motion zones from left to right: shoulder abduction, shoulder extension, and shoulder flexion.

When moving your shoulder up and down (flexion) or back and forth (abduction), keep your elbow in the green zone, which puts the least amount of stress on your shoulder. The yellow zone exerts moderate stress; use caution in this region. Whether in the green or yellow zone, make your motions efficient for activities, exercise, and rehabilitation. When you reach into the red zone, the shoulder is under the most stress, making it unstable and vulnerable to injury. Avoid motions in the red zones when possible, especially if you have an injured shoulder. The greater the range of motion, the more stress is placed on the joint. For movements in front of the body, if you can see your hands you are generally in the safe zone.

You can relate these zones to three kinds of shoulder/arm movements: opening your arms (abduction), lifting your arms forward (flexion), and taking your arms backward (extension). Note that each arm/shoulder may have a different comfort zone and that changing hand position (e.g., turning your palms up, facing them inward) can affect mobility in one or both shoulders.

To determine your zones when opening your arms (shoulder abduction), start by standing with your back against a wall.

1. Raise your arms in front of you at shoulder height with your palms facing each other. Now spread them to just where you can't see your hands anymore. Does this hurt? If not, this is your green zone—you can perform most activities in this zone and not hurt yourself.

2. Now spread your hands back to the wall. Does this hurt? This is the yellow zone—this is where some people display tightness. Whether or not you feel tightness, you should still be careful in this zone.

3. The red zone is behind you, such as when you reach into the back seat of the car without turning your body.

To determine your zones when moving your arms forward (shoulder flexion), start by standing with your arms alongside your body.

1. Raise your arms forward to shoulder height with your palms facing each other. This area should move freely and is your green zone.

2. As you raise your arms above shoulder height, you may feel some restriction. This is your yellow zone.

3. Anything above and beyond your head is the red zone.

To determine your zones when moving your arms backward (shoulder extension), start by standing with your arms alongside your body.

1. Slowly move your arms straight back 3–4 inches. This should feel relatively comfortable and is your green zone.

2. The difference between the yellow and red zones is very small, so be careful any time you move your arms back and up (to scratch your upper back, for instance).

SHOULDER BIOMECHANICS TIPS

By staying mindful of the following ways to perform proper shoulder biomechanics, you can dramatically reduce shoulder issues.

- Separate and lighten loads.

- Lift and carry loads close to your body.

- Take frequent breaks from any repetitious activity.

- Sleep on your back or your unaffected shoulder with a pillow between your arm and body. Watch that your shoulder stays in line with your body.

- Wear a fanny pack, sling your bag's strap across your body and unaffected shoulder, or tuck the load between your body and elbow.

- When performing shoulder-intensive activities like sweeping, vacuuming, and raking leaves, move your whole body by moving your feet, and keep your arm tucked in close to your side. Take small steps and keep your back straight.

- Use inexpensive "reachers" or grabber devices to protect your shoulder.

- Practice good posture.

- Rearrange your workstation.

- Alternate the arm with which you carry your briefcase or purse.

- Pay close attention to how your head and upper back are positioned at work and while doing daily activities.

- Minimize the load in your arms when sitting at your desk or workstation.

Avoid these activities:

- Don't slump and let your shoulders round forward.

- Don't perform prolonged overhead work.

- Don't work for more than 15–20 minutes without a rest break for your shoulder.

- Don't lift loads that are too heavy. Ask for assistance!

- Don't reach beyond your shoulder's safe (green) zone.

- Don't sleep on the affected shoulder.

- Don't sling your purse/briefcase over the affected shoulder.

- Don't rest on your affected arm while reading or watching TV.

- Don't carry heavy grocery bags—split the load.

- Don't stay in a prolonged "shrug/hunched over" posture such as having a phone between your ear and shoulder, being hunched over while texting, or carrying a purse. (Stand up regularly and stretch and do shoulder exercises.)

TRAINING SMART

Earlier we discussed that what you do today will have an impact on your shoulder health tomorrow. The following material is offered to shed some insights into that concept. This section identifies facts and myths about fitness and answers those questions that are most frequently asked. It will also provide a rationale for why some popular exercises fail the "benefit-to-risk" index. When they do fail the test, appropriate alternate exercises need to be included.

Everyone knows that physical activity and exercise is good for the human body. Unfortunately, in our zest to get fit, we often hurt ourselves because we're using outdated principles promoted by some overzealous trainer who has faulty assumptions. The computer industry has evolved over the past 20 years, and so has the understanding of the interplay of body mechanics and movement.

Some exercises have been around so long that it seems irreverent to question their efficacy. Successful coaches who have produced winning teams have passed down some faulty myths. Often, training methods get adopted and later institutionalized based on anecdotal information rather than science. And even what is scientifically acceptable today may change. Good sense suggests that even proper exercise, if done incorrectly, too quickly, or to an extreme, can be injurious to your health. Most of the exercise myths that we're going to discuss won't kill you today or even really hurt you if done once or twice. The problem is cumulative and manifests itself over time. The human body is very resilient, but if misused and abused, the negative effects of improper exercise will show up years later.

Our access to fitness videos and glitzy infomercials with air-brushed models leaves us all vulnerable to get-fit schemes. Most infomercials have just enough truth and facts in them to make them seem plausible. Couple that with your favorite fitness celebrity telling you that you can look like them in six weeks and it's no wonder that we fall for these get-fit-quick gimmicks. One expert stated that at least 90 percent of exercise programs include some exercises that are as detrimental as they are valuable. The key questions to ask when determining if an exercise is correct: Does it pass the benefit-to-risk ratio? Is this exercise doing more harm than good, and is there a safer, more effective way to get the desired results? Any exercise that has made it into your routine should give maximum return on your investment.

When you participate in a fitness routine or engage in a sport, ask yourself the following questions:

How do I feel while doing this exercise?

How do I feel after doing this exercise?

Do I know…

- Why I'm doing this exercise?

- If this movement may be causing long-term harm to my shoulder joint?

- If I'm performing this motion in a biomechanically correct manner?

If the answer is "no," reconsider what you're doing and why. Seek out professional advice if needed.

FIT TIPS

1. Not all trainers are equally qualified. If you come across a trainer who says, "No pain, no gain," RUN! If someone still subscribes to old-school and outdated concepts, RUN! Today, we maintain that the "no pain, no gain" concept is insane. As a former chief of surgery at a well-known teaching medical school told me, "While we can do remarkable things in surgery, we can never make the person as good as the original equipment. People need to take better care of themselves."

2. There are some biomechanical things to keep in mind when training.

- Be alert any time you raise your arms above your head.

- Doing lateral raises with your arms fully extended to the side can aggravate shoulder problems and may cause elbow problems as well. Also, there's a tendency to shrug the shoulders up near the ears when exercising the arms, so try to keep your shoulders relaxed when performing arm exercises.

- Keep proper upper-back posture when executing shoulder motions; ask a spotter to check your alignment or look in the mirror.

3. An important concept to keep in mind is not to become complacent about exercise or form in a sporting activity. It's critical to always be mindful of proper body mechanics when exercising or playing. Learn to listen to your body while working out. This means paying attention to what you're doing! While exercising may be boring, talking or listening to tunes can cause you to get careless in executing the movement properly. Only perfect practice makes perfect! Keep in mind that it takes many repetitions of executing a movement before it's ingrained into your muscle memory, so listening to music or talking distracts from that learning experience.

Remember the two-hour rule! If you hurt more two hours after your exercise session, you need to back off to a level that doesn't cause pain. If you continue to hurt or are losing range of motion, consult your doctor ASAP.

THE DANGEROUS DOZEN

The following exercises are considered controversial because they're part of most training programs but the trauma they may cause to the shoulder region is cumulative and may build up over time. As stated earlier, any exercise, if done incorrectly, can cause shoulder problems. But some common exercises are riskier than others. Any prolonged overhead movements, for instance, can contribute to shoulder impairments. Activities that include swimming the crawl stroke to painting ceilings, recreational activities such as serving a tennis ball, or even fitness activities in the weight room can contribute to a shoulder concern. Here are the unlucky 12 "shoulder slammers" you should be aware of:

1. Lat pull-downs that are performed behind the neck, done too quickly, or even pulled down far below chin level can cause issues to the shoulder joint. Another problem often seen with the lat pull-down is taking too wide of a grip. Note that performing wide-grip pull-ups or pull-ups behind the head can also agitate the shoulder.

2. Military presses done behind the head (pressing behind the neck) can lead to increased pressure on the shoulder joint and cervical spine as well as increased laxity of the soft tissues of the shoulder joint. Regular shoulder presses on machines if done wrong can contribute to the same issues as above; it's recommended that the seat is lowered to a less stressful position.

3. Dumbbell flys and reverse flys done to an extreme width into the yellow and red zones.

4. Bench presses with a wide grip on the barbell, dumbbells held too wide, or dropping the elbows too far down below or behind the bench can be stressful on the shoulder. Placing the hands in a more neutral grip puts less strain on the shoulder.

5. Lateral raises and frontal raises done too quickly or lifted to higher-than-shoulder height can contribute to impingement.

6. Upright rows could be potentially risky if the bar is pulled too high.

7. Shrugs done with improper grip width (too wide or too narrow) or letting the shoulders roll forward and drop quickly can set you up for a problem. Shrugs done properly with a comfortable weight are okay but engaging in non-weighted shrugs to improve scapular mobility is also a good idea.

8. As far as arm exercises on machines, bicep curls on a fixed bar can strain the shoulder joint. Instead, use a neutral grip. Avoid triceps machines or movements that require awkward positioning (e.g., French curls).

9. Bar dips done too low or too quickly can be problematic.

10. Push-ups done too wide or in a manner that strains your shoulder should be avoided. Push-ups done with hands in a neutral position are best.

11. Many boot camp–type exercises are often problematic and not correct for the average fitness participant. Even jumping jacks with improper shoulder force/movements can present a problem over time.

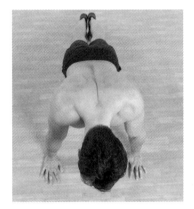

Neutral position

12. While water exercise is an excellent way to replicate weight training–type exercises, poor biomechanics and classes taught by ill-trained instructors can hurt you. When in the water, be mindful of the 3 S's: *size* of the object (hand vs. paddle), *speed* of the movement (fast vs. slow), and *shape* of the object (blunt vs. streamlined).

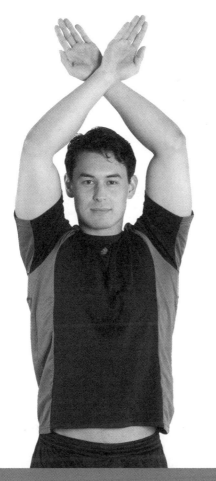

Part 2

CORRECTIVE EXERCISES

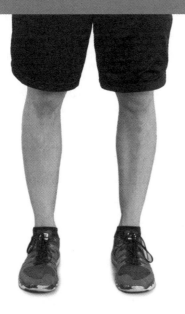

Chapter 4

SHOULDER REHABILITATION

Knowledge is power. To understand and commit to the rehabilitation process, you need to have to a basic understanding of your condition and the steps needed to fully recover. By most accounts, the shoulder joint is a difficult and complicated joint to rehabilitate.

With any dysfunction in the shoulder area, it's strongly advised that you see a health professional ASAP, especially if you have numbness in the hands and fingers or a loss of function. An early diagnosis followed with proper treatment improves your chances of a full and rapid recovery. Attempting to "play through" pain or dismissing your condition will only prolong your rehabilitation process. At the early stage of any dysfunction, the goal is to prevent further damage. At the first sign of a twinge in your shoulder, it's critical to ascertain the cause. Certain movements like overhead motions, sleeping on your affected side, or hanging your purse over your affected shoulder should be evaluated.

The three general stages of dysfunction are:

Mild—At this stage, the doctor may advocate a home-based exercise program that includes corrective exercise and specific stretches. Keep in mind, you're still injured, and re-injury is very common. Don't rush the body's healing.

Moderate—At this stage, passive, light, and active range-of-motion exercises may be recommended to prevent a frozen shoulder. Protective rest of the joint, as well as modalities to control pain, will be recommended.

Severe—In this stage, rest, ice, heat, and range-of-motion exercise are often recommended. In addition, pain management options such as medications or possible injections could be advised. Heat, whether through a hot bath or shower or applied via warm compress is generally okay for warming up the joint prior to corrective exercise. It often helps relieve stiffness and soreness but should not be used in an acute phase of injury.

SLEEPING WITH A FROZEN SHOULDER

A good night's sleep is when the body restores itself. Yet getting a good night's sleep when dealing with a chronic shoulder condition is often difficult. Some people even sleep in a recliner chair so as not to put pressure on the shoulder. Here are some tips for making bedtime more comfortable.

Back sleepers: Try placing your frozen shoulder on a pillow, and perhaps, placing a pillow under your knees. Your neck should not have excessive arch in it.

Side sleepers: Avoid sleeping directly on the affected shoulder. Sleep on your good side and place a pillow in front of you to rest your affected arm. Consider placing a pillow behind your knees to encourage proper sleep posture.

Stomach sleepers: Avoid sleeping on your stomach. It's not suggested for people with shoulder, back, or neck issues.

With early and proper intervention, shoulder function can be restored or minimally compromised. Before starting any type of rehabilitation work, it's wise to have a health professional perform a complete evaluation of both your active range of motion (your ability to move your joint on your own) and passive range of motion (the ability of your health care worker to move your joint). The health provider will compare the affected side to the unaffected side and then evaluate where the pain is coming from and why.

There are several options for the treatment of a frozen shoulder and other shoulder dysfunctions.

The pyramid on page 32 shows most invasive to least invasive.

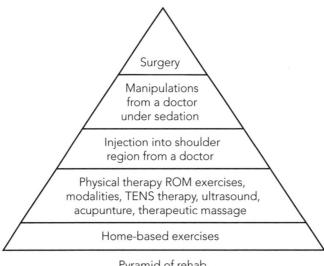

Pyramid of rehab

If you've tried a week of rest and self-help methods and your shoulder still isn't improving, it's time to seek medical advice and consider formalized therapy. Each therapist will have slightly different phases of "rehab." However, for the purpose of this book it will be kept rather basic. The doctor and therapist will guide you along the steps that are best for you and your condition. Often the treatment plan is different based on motivation and expected outcomes. For instance, the treatment plan for a major league pitcher will be different in scope and intensity than for most people. Your pain level and range of motion (ROM) are often key considerations.

There are three basic phases of rehabilitation for a frozen shoulder. In *Phase 1*, or the acute phase, the focus is to maintain and improve range of motion while addressing pain containment. The emphasis in *Phase 2*, the recovery phase, moves to improve joint stability. The focus should be on training the muscles closest to the joint that provide stability and support, such as the SITS muscles (subscapularis, supraspinatus, infraspinatus, and teres minor). The most important aspect in *Phase 3*, the functional phase, is improving functional fitness/work hardening, which prepares the joint for daily activities, such as work or recreational requirements.

Shoulder experts maintain that the timing at which each phase is introduced is the key to optimal recovery. Too much too soon is as bad as too little too late. Be patient. It may take six weeks or more to notice any improvement. Continue with your corrective exercises persistently until fully recovered. Even then it's wise to include corrective shoulder exercises post-injury.

Note: Since your health care provider is most familiar with the individual aspects of your condition, any information they provide supersedes any information discussed below. As you engage in any of the following programs, use pain as your guide.

The goal of a shoulder rehabilitation routine is to:

1. Decrease pain.

2. Do no further trauma to the area.

3. Improve range of motion.

4. Return to full restoration.

As you'll notice in the table below, the first phase highlights gentle, passive, and active range-of-motion "stretches" without an increase in stiffness or residual pain. In phase 2, you're trying to regain a functional and pain-free range of motion. The goal of phase 3 is to return you to your pre-injury status.

	GOALS
PHASE 1: ACUTE PHASE	• Managing pain • Maintaining range of motion • Maintaining neuromuscular control • Preventing muscle atrophy
PHASE 2: RECOVERY PHASE	• Preventing further injury and pain • Regaining upper-body strength and muscular balance and stability • Fostering shoulder flexibility • Improving neuromuscular control and coordination
PHASE 3 : FUNCTIONAL PHASE	• Improving functional fitness/work hardening that will prepare the joint for activities of daily living, whether at work or play

PHASE 1: ACUTE PHASE

The focus during Phase 1, also known as the acute phase or "freezing stage," is to maintain and improve range of motion while addressing pain containment. In the acute stage, the main focus is to do no further harm and hasten the healing process.

Training Tip: Always let your shoulder be your guide. Assess how you feel while doing the move and afterward.

Most experts suggest that mobility training precedes a strength-training routine. While training smart is always critical, it's most important at this stage. Being gentle with your joint is the operative word. Your shoulder is likely to be inflamed.

Phase 1 goals are:

- Managing pain

- Maintaining range of motion

- Maintaining neuromuscular control

- Preventing muscle atrophy

Phase 1 usually is the most painful. At this stage the medical doctor may suggest a course of NSAIDs and maybe rest, ice, or heat applications, as well as a series of formal physical therapy treatments. A trained therapist may apply ultrasound, or transcutaneous electrical nerve stimulation (TENS). A home program may be advised that consists of gently stretching of the shoulder capsule three times per day to keep the adhesions from getting too rigid, producing a "frozen shoulder." At this early stage of recovery, you should follow the exact orders of your health professional.

Phase 1 Sample Exercise Routine for Frozen Shoulder

PROGRESSION TO PHASE 2

When are you ready to move to the next level? Your shoulder will tell you. The pain level in your shoulder has decreased. (Don't overmedicate to mask pain.) You also have near-normal ROM and feel you can tolerate strength training. However, when in doubt, consult your health professional for clearance.

PHASE 2: RECOVERY PHASE

Phase 2 begins to address improving joint stability. Focus should be on training the muscles closest to the joint that provide stability and support, such as the SITS muscles (subscapularis, supraspinatus, infraspinatus, and teres minor).

In Phase 2, it's wise to continue with the Phase 1 mobility exercises. You can now consider adding a small weight to improve your capsular flexibility and adding some strengthening exercises to improve shoulder stability. Use pain as your guide. Continue performing a regular stretch session periodically throughout the day. Improving shoulder flexibility is the key to full restoration of the shoulder region.

Phase 2 goals are:

- Preventing further injury and pain

- Regaining upper-body strength and muscular balance and stability

- Fostering shoulder flexibility

- Improving neuromuscular control and coordination

Once you're given the okay by your health provider, start by selecting three to five exercises. The best method to determine which exercises are best for you to include is to try each exercise one or two times and see how your shoulder responds. Once you have decided which ones feel best for you, select three to five exercises for your routine and perform them for one to two weeks. After a couple weeks, once again test out which three to five exercises feel the best. Depending on how your shoulder reacts and how much time you have to perform the series, expand and adapt the routine to your specific characteristics. Generally, 15 minutes of corrective exercise is adequate. The reason that so many exercises are presented is to provide you a variety of options.

Progression Tip: Once you can do most of the exercises without an increase in pain or loss of function, consider progressing to Phase 3. If you have an increase in discomfort, return to the level you are comfortable with.

Phase 2 Sample Exercise Routine for Frozen Shoulder

Finger Walking (Frontal), page 60

Hanging Arm Circle, page 49

Forward & Backward Swing, page 47

PROGRESSION TO PHASE 3

The progression from one phase to the next is very subjective and based on your pain level and function. Some simple guideposts to whether you're ready to progress are: how you feel—there should be a decrease in pain without an increase in medication; a decrease of pain two hours after exercise as well as the next day; and an improvement in range of motion. Consult with your doctor if you have any doubts.

PHASE 3: FUNCTIONAL PHASE

The emphasis in this stage, also known as the thawing level, is to return your shoulder to "normal" functional ability. By this stage you understand what level of strength and flexibility you need to perform your daily duties. You need to evaluate what *your* normal is to function. While "normal" for an uninjured shoulder may be 180 degrees of flexion, you may need less than that to perform your activities of daily living. Also, normal for a professional athlete is much different than the average office worker. You need to critically evaluate the amounts of muscular strength, endurance, and/or flexibility that are reasonably needed for your personal needs.

If you've been suffering with a frozen shoulder for a significant amount of time, your shoulder and arm region may have significantly atrophied. You may need to strengthen your weakened shoulder muscles, so take it gently. Most frozen shoulder patients are able to redevelop their muscle strength just by resuming their normal everyday activities. However, taking a proactive approach by participating in corrective exercises may hasten your full and functional recovery.

Engaging in too much too soon will only contribute to a setback in your recovery. To avoid a relapse, evaluate your activities, recreational pursuits, body mechanics, and posture to see if they could've been the culprits in the development of your condition. Consider including corrective postural exercises. Too often people adopt a protective posture to relieve pain or perform a required function. Ask your physical therapist or human resources officer at work to bring in an ergonomics professional to evaluate your workstation.

Phase 3 goal is:

Improving functional fitness/work hardening that will prepare the joint for activities of daily living, whether at work or play. Learn to listen to your body. If anything hurts—stop!

Once you're given the okay by your health care provider, select two to five exercises to perform from the Phase 3 exercises below. As you progress, add and omit exercises as you desire. Your exercise program should be a living document that adapts to your goals and ability. Prior to exercise, remember to warm up the region with moist heat. Some shoulder experts have found that performing Hanging Arm Circles and Graduated Presses will help. These exercises involve either using a small 1kg weight or a resistance band. These should only be performed when pain has diminished more than 90 percent.

Phase 3 Sample Exercise Routine for Frozen Shoulder

Corner Stretch, page 93

Graduated Press, page 112

END OF PHASE 3

The end of Phase 3 is somewhat arbitrary. You should sincerely feel that you've come a long way in your recovery and are ready for full engagement in your life. However, if you push yourself too hard now, you can easily cause a relapse. Take your time—remember how you felt before and how long it took to recover. You should feel as if you have the ability to return to pre-injury activities and, as silly as this sounds, you can do "normal" activities and forget that you had a difficult time performing them weeks ago. If you think you're ready—congratulations! Now it's time to move on to strength and conditioning exercises that will help you avoid reinjury. See Part 3 for tips on how to create an ongoing program that will strengthen your shoulder and maintain shoulder health.

Chapter 5

PHASE 1, 2, AND 3 EXERCISES

The purpose of this section is to provide you with a comprehensive array of shoulder exercises, stretches, and movements for every phase of your recovery. Every effort was made to include only movements and exercises that are recognized by shoulder experts and therapists to be most advantageous for a frozen shoulder and shoulder injuries. The focus of the exercises in this section is to do no harm while providing the most benefits and the least amount of risk. Keep in mind that not every exercise is correct for every person or every condition.

HOW TO USE THIS SECTION

It's highly recommended that you take this book to your health professional and ask them to highlight which exercises would be best for you. In this way, this book could be much like having a personal coach assist you with your recovery. Ask the health professional to personalize the program for you with regard to the number of times you should perform the exercises and for how many weeks, then check in again after a few weeks to have them add or delete certain exercises. Most health professionals will applaud your proactive approach that will complement your therapy and facilitate your recovery. Note that none of these exercises is a silver bullet to recovery. Exercise therapy is much like every aspect of medicine—a combination of art and science. If something isn't working, consult your health professional for a little tweaking of your treatment plan. Most importantly, listen to your shoulder—it will tell you which exercises are correct for you!

The exercises in each phase were grouped by difficulty, from easiest to most challenging and include those done while sitting, standing, or lying on the floor. However, everyone's body is different, so allow your body to "coach" you. Don't make pain! Most exercises duplicate function so you can simply replace and insert different exercises based on your motivation and pain tolerance. Additionally, some of the exercises are of equal difficulty, but, in reality, only you will be able to understand which is easiest based on your tolerance to the exercise. You're the captain of the ship—adapt according to how the exercise feels and how you respond.

Depending on your pathophysiology and diagnosis, certain movements will be best for you. Treat this book as a smorgasbord of shoulder exercises and pick those that are best for you. Consult with your health professional if you are unsure about any exercises you aren't sure about for your specific condition.

Fit Tip: Remember, more isn't always better and only by doing the movements correctly will your condition improve. Only perfect practice makes perfect. Keep in mind that pain is your body's early-alert system, so listen to it.

Important note: The information given by your health professional supersedes any information provided in this book because they're familiar with your unique situation.

Recovery of your shoulder may take weeks or even months depending on your diagnosis or the severity of problem. In the game of shoulder rehabilitation, slow and steady wins the race. Progressing too quickly will only set you up for re-injury. As you embark on the recovery process, you need to become your own personal trainer. The goal of a good trainer is to do no harm. Avoid any activity that aggravates your shoulder. Never mask your pain with pills or lotions. Pain is your body's way of informing you that something bad is going on. To prevent a re-injury or unnecessary pain, execute motions within a pain-free zone with proper form. If you suspect a re-injury, schedule a follow-up appointment with your doctor ASAP.

Setting time each day to focus on proper execution of each movement will hasten recovery. Prior to performing these motions, warm up the area first with a warm shower, a moist heat pack, or light activity. Consult with your health care provider first as to how you should warm up the joint. Most importantly, listen to your body and heed what it says. If it says, "I am fatigued," don't force one more repetition. If it says, after a workout, "I hurt!" back off. Keep in mind the two-hour rule: If your shoulder hurts more two hours post-exercise, back off until you're pain-free.

The proper application of heat and ice is an important factor to consider in your treatment plan. The general rule of thumb is use heat prior to exercise and ice after completion of your routine. Speak with your doctor/therapist about how and when they want you to apply heat and/or ice. Use caution and good sense when applying heat to the area to avoid a burn.

WORKOUT TIPS

In addition to gently moving your shoulder several times each day, aim to perform your selected exercises three times a day, such as in the morning after a shower, mid-day while on your lunch break, and sometime in the evening, perhaps after a shower. Most experts suggest to work up to holding each static stretch 15–60 seconds. If you can treat the session like a yoga class with soft lighting and mellow music that won't distract you from focusing on the biomechanics of the movement, perhaps the session will feel like retreat time rather than drudgery. When engaging in the exercises, focus on healthy deep breaths as well as mindful movements. The general guideline for deep breathing is a 1:2 ratio, which might be a two-second inhalation through the nose and a four-second exhalation through the mouth.

- Never overmedicate prior to exercising to mask pain. Most doctors suggest that if you're on medication (NSAIDs, for instance), select an exercise time when the medication is having its maximum effect.

- To improve blood flow to the region, take a couple of minutes to do a little aerobic exercise, such as jogging in place, prior to engaging in any shoulder motions.

- Maintain proper posture. Try performing exercises in front of a mirror for feedback.

- Apply heat/warmth to involved area prior to exercise. Use cold on the affected shoulder area post-exercise if desired.

- Don't make pain. If you experience any increase in pain or symptoms, don't continue with any exercise and consult with your health care provider.

If you notice any new symptoms such as pain, numbness, or tingling, see your health care provider.

PHASE 1 EXERCISES

The following exercises are listed in almost every publication reviewed as acceptable beginning exercises for people suffering from frozen shoulder. Note that you don't need to perform every exercise. Some exercises duplicate goals and objectives so select those that feel best. The goal of this section is to prevent the shoulder from becoming frozen. It's also prudent to tackle a small problem early and get on top of it before it progresses to a major issue. The exercises in this section can be used in either case. If you desire, you may perform any of these exercises on both sides. Select two to three exercises to perform; as you progress, add and delete exercises as you desire.

As you improve, and with medical approval, consider adding a light weight to the standing exercises. Note that the weight is not intended for strength building, only to provide traction.

GOAL: to gently improve range of motion

TARGET: shoulder joint

Start with this passive exercise before you add any weights. Apply warmth and perform this exercise gently. It's very simple but easy to get wrong so please follow the instructions carefully.

1 Bend forward at the waist and let the affected arm hang toward the floor under its own weight. Feel the sense of tugging and traction in the shoulder joint. If helpful, you can support your other hand on a chair.

2 Move your body to make the hanging arm swing gently. Use this method to swing or rock the arm in small-to medium-sized circles.

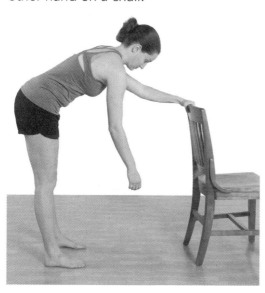

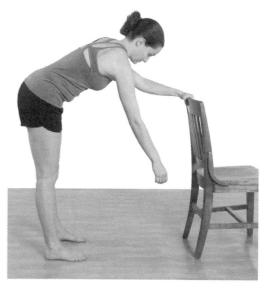

You may want to ice your shoulder after this series of movements and assess how you feel before continuing.

SHOULDER SHRUG

GOAL: mobility to shoulder region

TARGET: trapezius muscle

Frozen shoulder sufferers can perform shoulder shrugging 5 times daily for 1–2 minutes. You can move both shoulders at the same time and then independently, but be careful if you have any neck problems.

1 Stand upright.

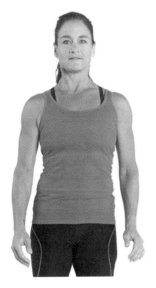

2 Shrug your shoulders upward as high as you can for 8 seconds.

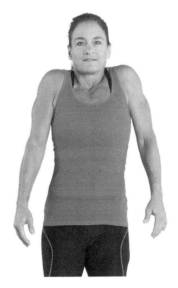

Let your shoulders drop to the start position.

Repeat 3 times.

GOAL: improve shoulder mobility

TARGET: trapezius

This can also be performed while sitting, or while taking a warm shower. Do not perform this exercise until you feel comfortable doing Shoulder Shrugs (page 44).

1 Stand with proper posture. Inhale slowly and deeply through your nose.

2 Exhaling through your nose, roll your shoulders forward, attempting to touch your shoulders together.

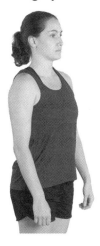

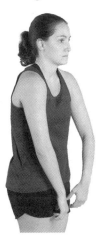

3 Inhale and move your shoulders back as you squeeze your shoulder blades together, opening up your chest.

VARIATION

If you can do this comfortably, try moving your shoulders in circular motions both forward and backward.

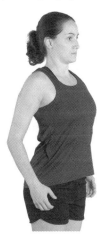

Repeat as desired.

SHOULDER BOX

GOAL: improve shoulder mobility

TARGET: trapezius

This can also be performed while sitting, or while taking a warm shower. Do not perform this exercise until you feel comfortable doing Shoulder Rolls (page 44).

1 Stand with proper posture.

2 Inhaling slowly and deeply through your nose, shrug your shoulders up.

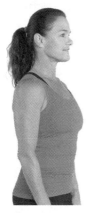

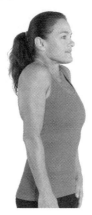

3 Exhaling through your lips, squeeze your shoulder blades together as you slowly lower them back down to start position.

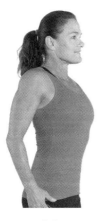

At the completion of the exercise, you have outlined the shape of a box.

Repeat as desired.

GOAL: improve shoulder range of motion

TARGET: shoulder

This could be done while taking a warm shower.

1 While standing, place the unaffected arm on a solid object and lean over at the waist.

2–3 Gently swing the affected arm back and forth alongside your body. Start with small swings and increase the size of the swings over time. Allow gravity to pull your arm down, and use your shoulder muscles to do the work, not your arm.

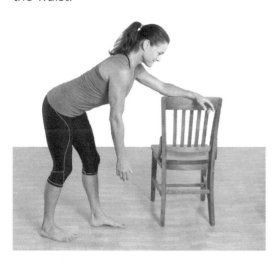

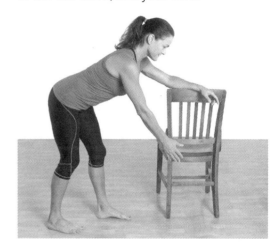

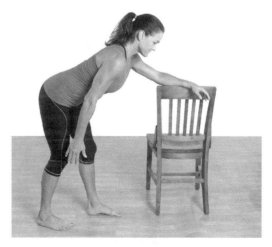

Repeat as desired.

CROSS-BODY SWING

GOAL: increase adduction and abduction range of motion of shoulder

TARGET: shoulder

This could be done while taking a warm shower. Be careful not to slip.

1 While standing, place the unaffected arm on a solid object and lean over at the waist.

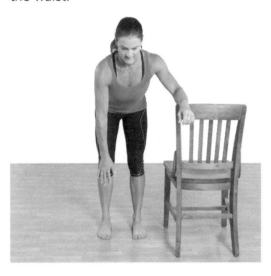

2–3 Gently swing the affected arm across your body, gradually increasing the width of your swings. Allow gravity to pull your arm down, and use your shoulder muscles to do the work, not your arm.

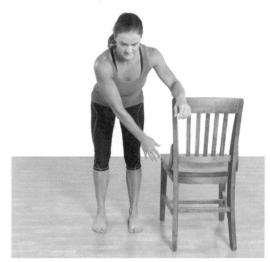

VARIATION

As you improve, and with medical approval, consider adding a light weight or a soup can.

Repeat as desired.

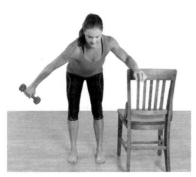

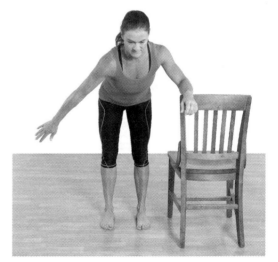

GOAL: increase shoulder range of motion

TARGET: shoulder

This could be done while taking a warm shower. Be careful not to slip.

1 While standing, place the unaffected arm on a solid object and lean over at the waist.

2 Gently swing the affected arm in a small clockwise direction. Allow gravity to pull your arm down, and use your shoulder muscles to do the work, not your arm. Start with small swings and increase the size of the swings over time.

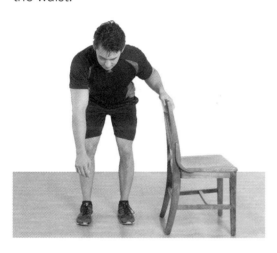

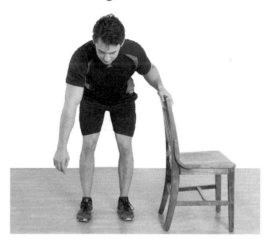

3 Gently swing arm in small counterclockwise direction.

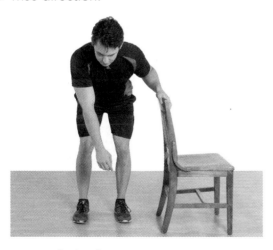

VARIATION

As you improve, and with medical approval, consider adding a light weight or a soup can.

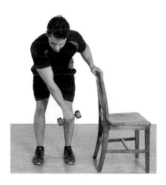

Repeat as desired.

WOOD CHOP

GOAL: increase shoulder flexion range of motion

TARGET: shoulder

1 Stand with proper posture. Position your hands in front of your body and interlace your fingers.

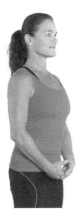

2 Keeping your arms straight, slowly raise both arms as high as possible. Don't arch your back to gain additional range of motion. It's okay for your uninjured arm/shoulder to assist the frozen shoulder arm.

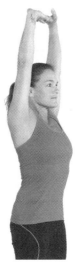

Slowly lower arms to start position.

Repeat as desired.

LYING VARIATION

Lie on your back. Allow adequate time for your chest and shoulder region to relax and open up. Breathe naturally and get comfortable. Once comfortable and stable, interlace your fingers and extend both arms up toward ceiling; use your unaffected arm to assist. Once comfortable, drop both hands backward toward the floor, leading with your thumbs. Stay within your pain-free range of motion.

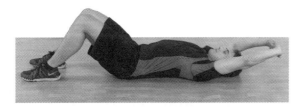

GOAL: improve functional range of motion

TARGET: shoulder

THE POSITION: Stand with your back against a wall and reach your affected arm up the wall as tolerated. Feel the stretch through the shoulder area and relax and breathe freely. You can also do this by facing the wall and reaching up to a comfortable height.

ADVANCED VARIATION

To achieve a more pronounced stretch, slightly bend your knees to lower your body. Keep the arm in the extended position. Only squat to a depth that stretches the area but doesn't strain.

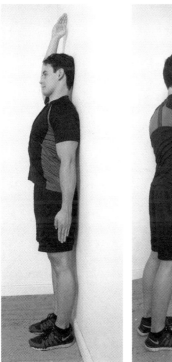
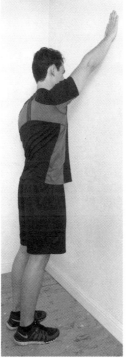
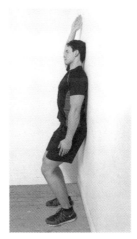
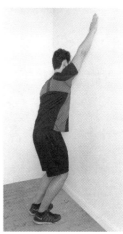

CROSS-SHOULDER TOUCH

GOAL: increase adduction and abduction range of motion of the shoulder

TARGET: shoulder

This can also be performed while standing.

1 Sit with proper posture in a stable chair with your arms alongside your body.

2 Using the hand of the injured shoulder, reach across your chest and attempt to touch your opposite shoulder.

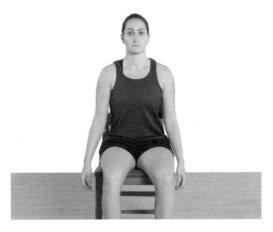

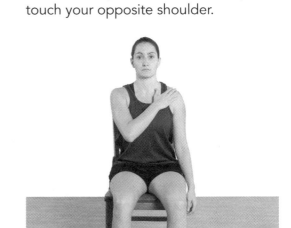

3 Return to start position and then reach behind your head to touch the opposite shoulder.

Repeat as desired.

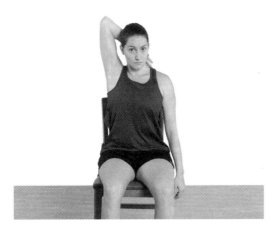

Return to start position.

GOAL: increase shoulder range of motion

TARGET: shoulder girdle

Some shoulder experts suggest placing a towel on a smooth surface to facilitate ease of motion. If need be, use your unaffected arm to place your injured arm on table.

1 Sit at a table and place your affected forearm on the table.

2 Straighten your arm by slowly reaching across the table. Hold for 5–10 seconds.

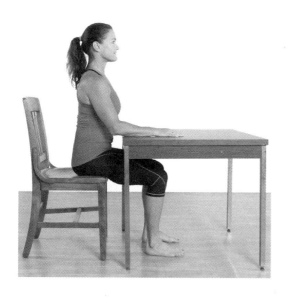
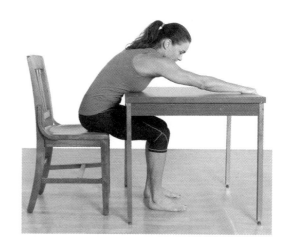

Return to start position.

Repeat as desired.

MODIFICATION

If you have a severely frozen shoulder, use the motion of leaning back to "pull" your arm back to start position. Essentially, your arm isn't doing the work. As you improve, utilize the arm and shoulder muscles more.

ARM SWING FLEXION/EXTENSION

GOAL: improve functional mobility

TARGET: shoulder girdle

1 Lie on your back. Allow adequate time for your chest and shoulder region to relax and open up. Breathe naturally and get comfortable.

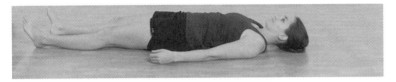

2 Raise both arms upward.

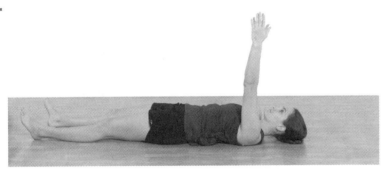

3 Move one arm forward and the other arm backward, within a safe range of motion.

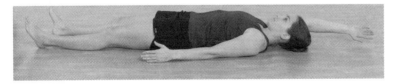

Perform the rhythmic motion for 30–60 seconds or as tolerated.

GOAL: increase shoulder range of motion

TARGET: shoulder girdle

1 Lie on your back. Allow adequate time for your chest and shoulder region to relax and open up. Breathe naturally and get comfortable.

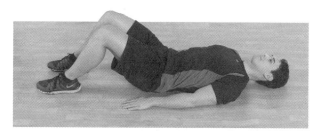

2 Place the hand of your frozen shoulder under the armpit of the opposite shoulder.

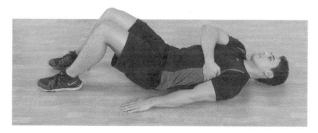

3 Place the hand of your unaffected shoulder on the elbow of your injured arm and gently press the elbow of the frozen shoulder toward the floor. Don't roll your torso. Hold for a comfortable moment.

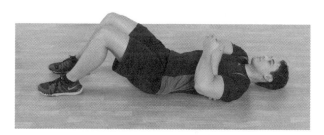

SUPINE SHOULDER PRESS

GOAL: foster shoulder range of motion and chest flexibility

TARGET: shoulder, chest

1 Lying on your back with your knees bent, grasp a cane or stick with each hand shoulder-width apart at chest level.

2 Press the cane up toward the ceiling, extending your arms fully if possible.

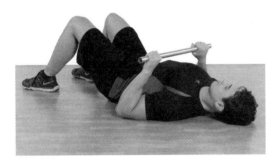

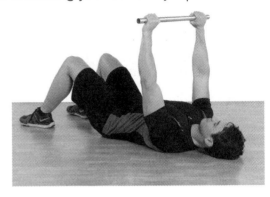

Return to start position.

Repeat as desired.

PROGRESSION

As you improve, add a light weight; perhaps attach a light sandbag securely across the cane. Be careful it doesn't fall on you.

GOAL: foster shoulder range of motion

TARGET: shoulder girdle

1 Lying on your back with your knees bent, grasp a cane or stick with each hand shoulder-width apart at chest level.

PROGRESSION

As you improve, add a light weight; perhaps attach a light sandbag securely across the cane. Be careful it doesn't fall on you.

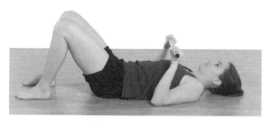

2 Press the cane up toward the ceiling, extending your arms fully if possible.

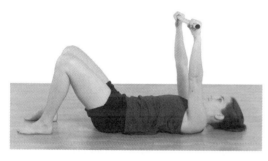

3 Keeping your arms straight, slowly allow your hands to drop as far back toward the floor as comfortable. Don't allow your lower back to arch.

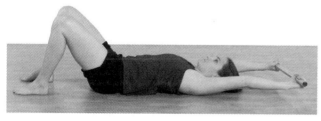

Return to start position.

Repeat as desired.

SUPINE LATERAL DROP WITH CANE

GOAL: increase range of motion

TARGET: chest, shoulder

1 Lying on your back with your knees bent, grasp a cane or stick with each hand shoulder-width apart at chest level.

2 Press the cane up toward the ceiling, extending your arms fully if possible.

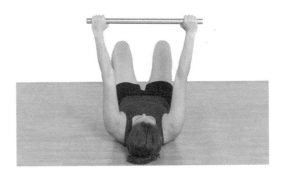

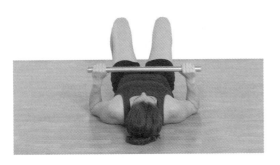

3 Keeping your arms straight, slowly drop the cane to one side as far as is comfortable.

4 Return to center and then drop to the opposite side.

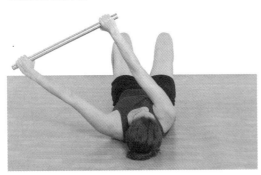

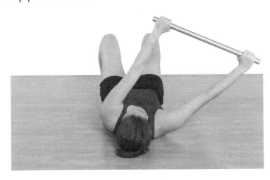

Return to start position.

Repeat as desired.

GOAL: increase range of motion and stabilization of shoulder

TARGET: shoulder girdle

1 Lie on your back. Allow adequate time for your chest and shoulder region to relax and open up. Breathe naturally and get comfortable.

2 Once comfortable and stable, extend both arms up toward the ceiling as high as is comfortable, using your unaffected arm to assist if necessary.

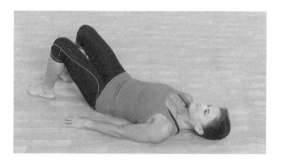

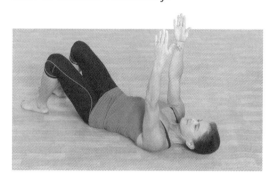

3 When comfortable using the involved arm, pretend to write your name, alphabet, etc., on the ceiling. Keep the unaffected arm on the floor. Stay within your pain-free zone. As you progress, allow the frozen arm/shoulder to increase its range of motion.

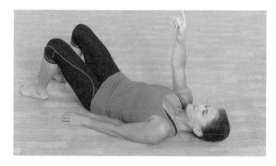

Repeat as desired.

PHASE 2 EXERCISES

The goal of this series is to improve functional range of motion. Start with two to five exercises, evaluate how they feel, and then add or delete exercises as you wish. The following exercises can be done on both the affected and unaffected sides.

FINGER WALKING (FRONTAL)

GOAL: increase shoulder flexion, range of motion, and functional ability

TARGET: shoulder

This can also be done while taking a warm shower.

1 Stand facing a wall about an arm's length away. With the fingertips of your affected arm, touch the wall at shoulder level.

2 Slowly walk your fingers up the wall as high as is comfortable. Don't arch your back or twist your body to gain height.

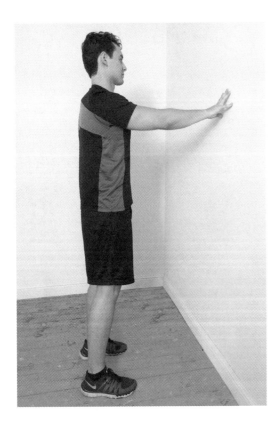

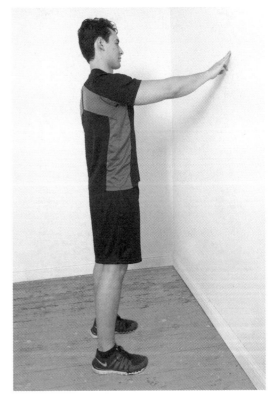

Return to start position.

Repeat as desired.

GOAL: increase abduction of shoulder joint and functional ability

TARGET: shoulder

This can also be done while taking a warm shower.

1 Stand sideways to a wall about an arm's length away. With the fingertips of your affected arm, touch the wall just below shoulder level.

2 With your arm outstretched, slowly allow your fingertips to walk up the wall as high as is tolerated. Don't lean or elevate your shoulder to gain additional height.

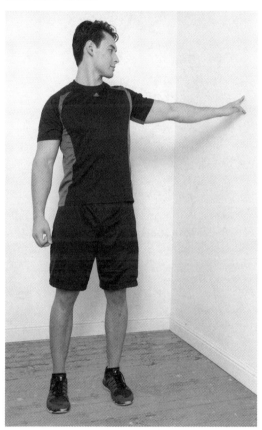

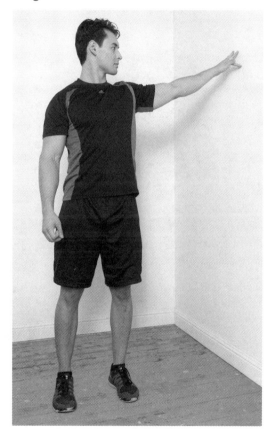

Return to start position.

Repeat as desired.

SIDE WALL CIRCLES

GOAL: increase flexion/extension and functional ability

TARGET: shoulder

1 Stand sideways with your affected shoulder an arm's length away from the wall. Extend your arm and touch the wall with a fingertip.

2 Begin drawing small circles clockwise, gradually increasing the size of the circles.

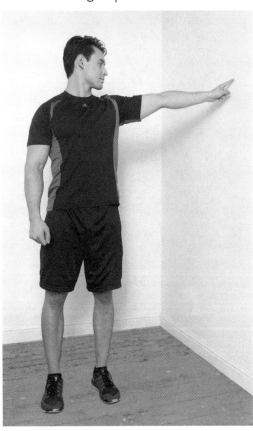

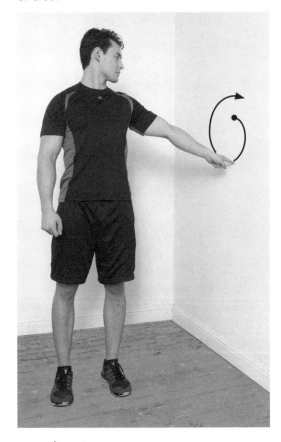

Reverse direction.

Repeat as desired.

GOAL: increase shoulder mobility rotation

TARGET: shoulder

1 Stand facing a wall about an arm's length away. With the fingertips of your affected arm, touch the wall at shoulder level.

2 Slowly draw a small circle clockwise. As you feel comfortable, make increasingly larger circles.

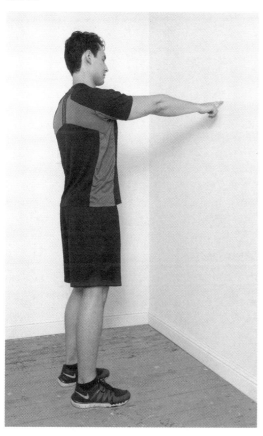

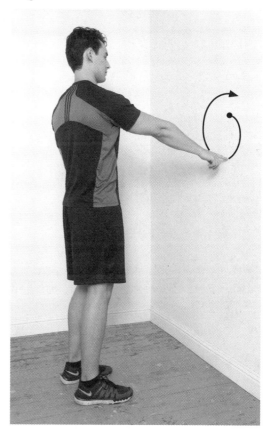

Reverse directions, making small circles that progress to larger ones.

Repeat as desired.

APPLE PICKER

GOAL: increase joint mobility and functional ability

TARGET: shoulder

1 Stand with proper posture and place your hands on your shoulders.

2 Reach your right hand to the ceiling as high as is comfortable.

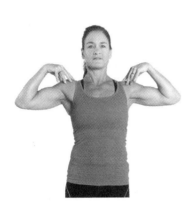

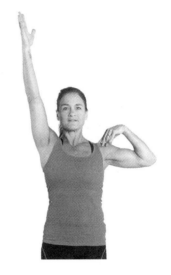

3 Place the right hand back on your shoulder. Now reach up with your left hand.

VARIATION

You can also try to touch your hand to the back of each shoulder and then the front of each shoulder.

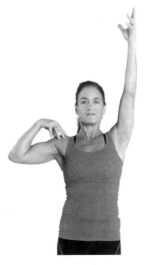

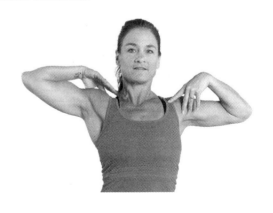

Repeat as desired, staying within your pain-free zone.

GOAL: warm up and improve posture

TARGET: chest, shoulder retractor

1 Lie on your back with your knees bent and feet flat on the floor. Clasp your hands behind your head.

2 Slowly bring your elbows together in front of your body.

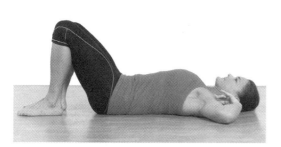

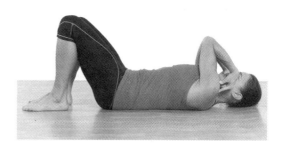

3 Now take your elbows out to the sides while squeezing your shoulder blades together. Hold for a moment, focusing on opening up your chest.

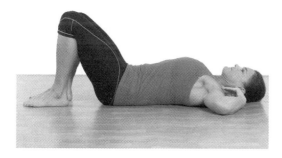

Return to start position.

Repeat as desired.

RESCUE ME

GOAL: increase scapular mobility and functional ability

TARGET: shoulder

1 Standing with proper position, raise both arms arm out to the sides into a "T" position.

2 Attempting to keep your shoulder blades down and in a locked position, raise your arms straight above your head if possible. This motion resembles a drowning victim signaling for help.

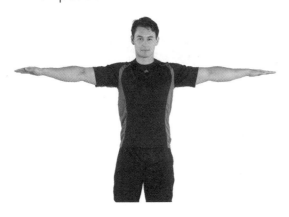

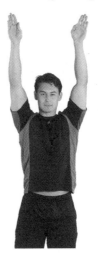

3 Lower your arms to the "T" position, focusing on shoulder blade placement.

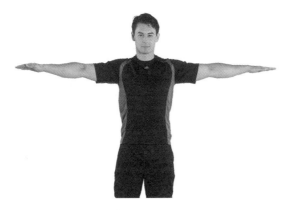

Repeat as desired.

VARIATION 1

With both arms extended along your sides and palms forward, raise your arms as high as possible and cross your wrists at the top.

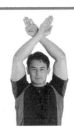

VARIATION 2

From the "T" position, stretch your arms out to the sides and cross your arms in front of your chest if possible.

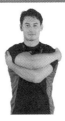

GOAL: increase shoulder flexion and functional ability

TARGET: shoulder

1 Stand with proper posture with your arms alongside your body. Turn your thumbs up.

2 Keeping your arms straight, raise your arms as high as possible, as if signaling a touchdown. Remember to keep your shoulder blades under control. Lower your arms slowly.

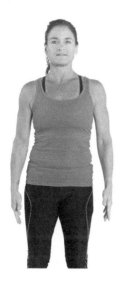

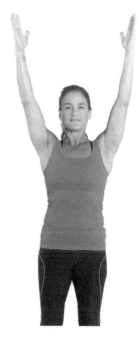

Repeat as desired.

VARIATION

This exercise can also be done while lying on the floor.

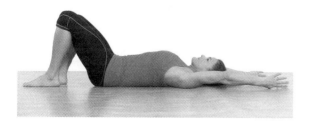

CHOKER

GOAL: improve shoulder flexibility

TARGET: rotator cuff

This stretch can also be done while taking a warm shower or sitting at your desk.

1 Stand with proper posture and place the hand of your affected shoulder on your unaffected shoulder.

2 Place the hand of your unaffected shoulder on the elbow of your affected shoulder and gently press the arm of your affected shoulder toward your throat. Hold the position for a comfortable moment.

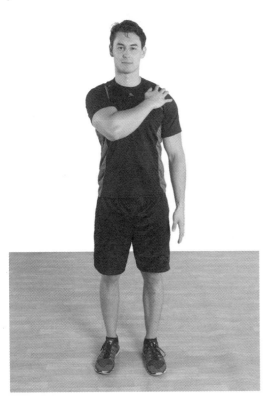

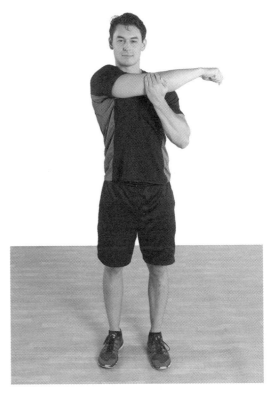

Switch sides and repeat.

GOAL: improve shoulder functional mobility and internal rotation

TARGET: shoulder

This can be performed while standing or sitting.

1 Stand with good posture and place the hand of your affected shoulder on your unaffected shoulder.

2–3 Slowly try to touch your hand to each rear pocket, alternating left and right rear pockets if possible. Return to start position.

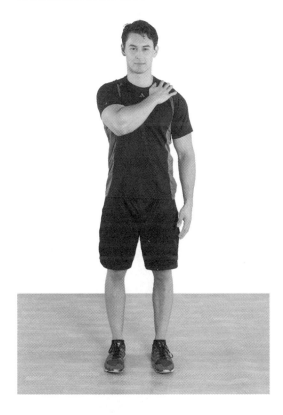
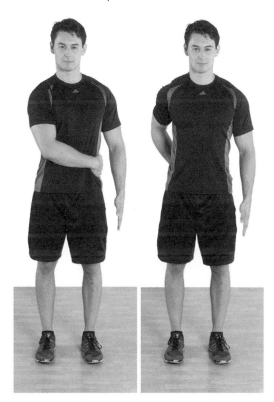

Repeat as desired.

TOWEL STRETCH

GOAL: increase shoulder flexibility

TARGET: rotator cuff

This can be uncomfortable so proceed with caution. Don't try this exercise until the above exercises can be done with no undue concern. This stretch can also be done while seated. If this is too painful or your shoulder is too stiff, don't perform. Consider icing after this move.

1 Stand with proper posture. While holding on to a towel/strap/belt with your affected hand, throw or drape a small towel/strap/belt over your frozen shoulder and down your back, grasping the towel behind your back with your good hand wherever you can reach it comfortably. Hold the position for a comfortable moment.

2 When and if you're ready, VERY gently pull the towel upward toward the sky. Perform as tolerated to a comfortable outstretched arm position and hold as tolerated up to 10 seconds.

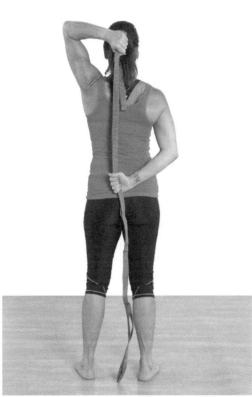

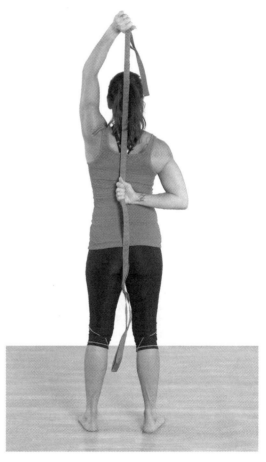

Repeat as tolerated and then switch arm positions.

GOAL: increase shoulder flexibility

TARGET: rotator cuff

Once you can perform the Towel Stretch (page 70), perform the following with caution. Don't try this until the above exercises can be done with no undue concern. This stretch can be done while standing in a warm shower or sitting at your desk.

1 Stand with proper posture. Reach behind your head and down your back with the hand of your affected shoulder. Your fingertips will be down and your palm will be toward back.

2 Place the hand of your unaffected shoulder on your other elbow and gently press the arm down your back. Hold the position for a comfortable moment.

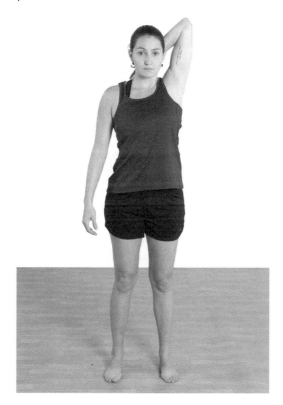

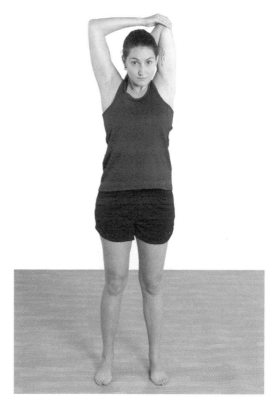

Repeat as desired.

UP THE BACK

GOAL: increase shoulder flexibility and internal rotation

TARGET: rotator cuff

Once you can perform the Towel Stretch (page 70), perform the following with caution. Don't try until the above exercises can be done with no undue concern. This stretch can be done while sitting or in a warm shower.

1 Stand with proper posture and move the hand of your frozen shoulder to the small of your back with your palm facing outward.

2 Place the hand of your unaffected shoulder on your other wrist/hand and gently press your arm up your back as far as feels comfortable. Hold the position for a comfortable moment. If your shoulder is too painful or too stiff, don't perform this.

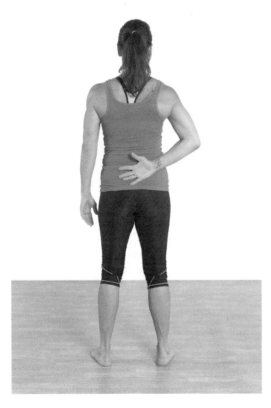

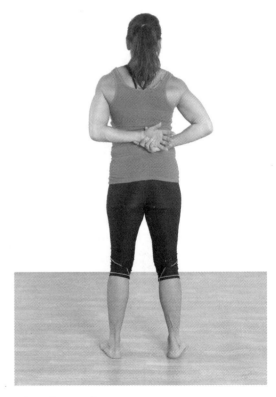

Switch sides and repeat.

GOAL: increase shoulder external rotation

TARGET: chest

1 Stand in a doorway and place each hand on either side of the doorframe.

2 Slowly take 1 step forward and gently find a comfortable stretch in the shoulder/chest region. Hold as tolerated. If the movement is too difficult, avoid it.

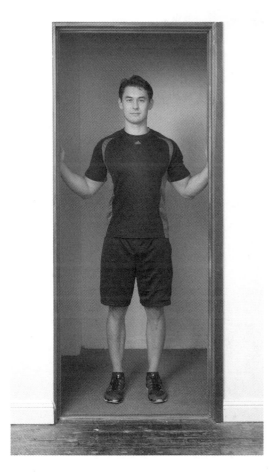

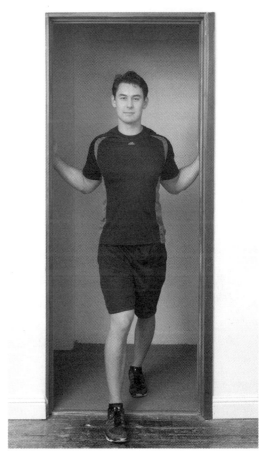

Repeat as desired.

CANE PRESS

GOAL: increase functional shoulder range of motion and flexibility

TARGET: shoulder

This can also be performed while sitting.

1 Standing with proper posture, hold a cane or stick with both hands at shoulder level, palms forward.

2 Press the cane upward as high as is comfortable. It's okay to press up at an angle to reduce any stress in your shoulder joints, but avoid arching your back to increase height.

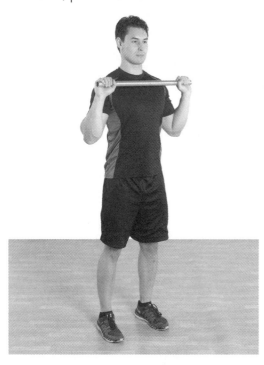

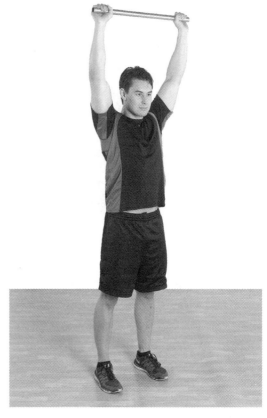

Return to start position.

Repeat as desired.

VARIATION

For an extra challenge, drape a sandbag across the cane.

GOAL: increase shoulder range of motion and function flexibility

TARGET: shoulder

This can also be performed while sitting.

1 Standing with proper posture, hold a cane or stick with both hands shoulder-width apart, palms facing down. Bend your elbows 90 degrees and keep them close to your torso. You can place a pillow or small rolled-up towel between your body and arm for comfort.

2–3 Keeping your torso stationary, slowly move the cane left and right, staying within your pain-free zone.

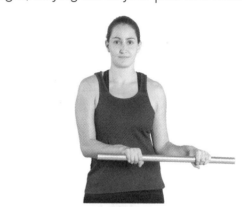

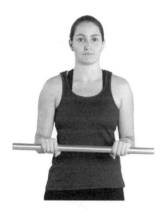

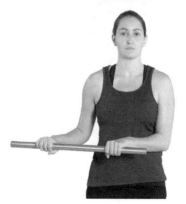

MODIFICATION

You can also perform this with both palms up or one palm up, one palm down.

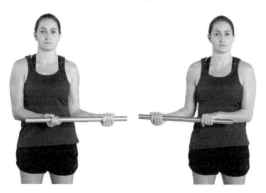

PHASE 3 EXERCISES

Before commencing with the exercises in this section, obtain permission from your health professional. The goal of this section is to improve your functional range of motion. Additionally, the exercises in this section could be used as preventive exercises as well as pre-workout warm-ups or post-exercise active stretches. It's a good idea to do these exercises with both the affected and unaffected shoulders as a preventive measure. Start with two to five exercises, evaluate how they feel, and then add or delete exercises as you wish.

SHOULDER PROGRESS APPRAISAL

1 Stand with proper posture and hold a ruler in one hand, placing your fingertips at the 12-inch mark. Reach that arm behind your head with the ruler tip down.

2 Now move your other hand behind your back and see how high you can reach. Ask someone to measure your score.

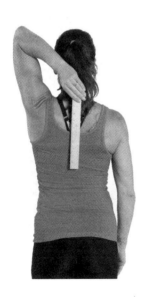

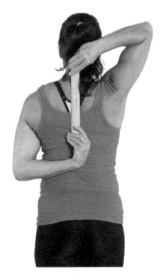

Repeat on the other side. Are the results the same? Keep the results and re-measure periodically to see if you are improving. Ideally you like both arms to have the same score.

GOAL: increase shoulder girdle flexibility and improve posture

TARGET: shoulder, chest

This can also be performed while sitting. Each time you do this exercise, subjectively or objectively measure if your pain-free range of motion is improving.

1 Stand with proper posture and place your hands behind your head.

2 Slowly move your elbows backward while bringing your shoulder blades together. The focus is on opening up your chest and tightening the upper-back muscles. Only go as far back as is comfortable. Hold for a moment.

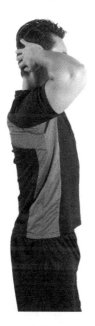

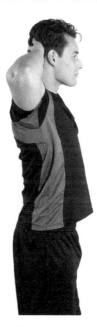

Repeat as desired.

VARIATION

You can perform this with your back and head against the wall for feedback. Aim to touch your elbows to the wall.

PICTURE FRAME

GOAL: increase shoulder mobility

TARGET: shoulder

This can also be performed while sitting.

1 Stand with proper posture. Place your right hand on your left elbow and your left hand on your right elbow.

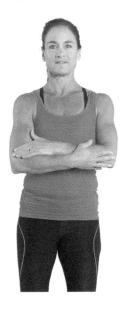

2 Slowly raise your arms overhead, lifting your arms only as high as feels comfortable. You're now framing your face in a picture frame created by your arms—smile! Hold the position for a moment, staying mindful of proper posture and not arching your lower back.

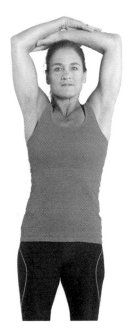

Repeat as desired.

VARIATION

You can perform this with your back and head against the wall for feedback.

GOAL: increase shoulder range of motion

TARGET: shoulder

This can also be done while standing with your back to a wall.

1 Lie on the floor with your arms at your sides, palms facing upward. If this is not possible, STOP. You're not ready for this exercise.

2 Keeping your knuckles on the floor, inhale deeply through your nose and sweep your arms until they're beside your ears or as close as is comfortable.

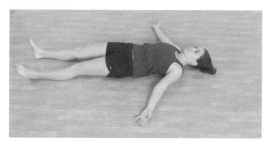

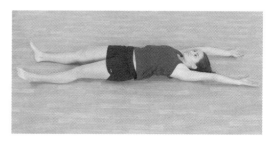

3 Exhale and slowly return your arms by your sides.

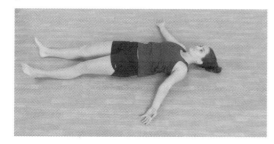

MODIFICATION

This exercise can also be done one arm at a time.

Repeat as desired.

SHOULDER BLADE SQUEEZE

GOAL: strengthen upper-back muscles, improve posture, and improve stabilizer muscles of the upper back

TARGET: upper back

1 Stand with proper posture.

2 Focusing on contracting the muscles between your shoulder blades, attempt to place your hands behind your tail-bone. Be careful not to arch your lower back or allow your neck and head to drop forward. Hold for 3–5 seconds.

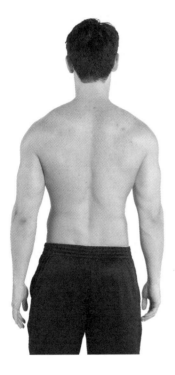

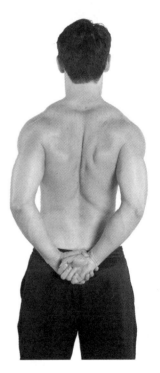

Relax.

Repeat as desired.

GOAL: improve posture

TARGET: shoulder joint stabilizer muscles

1 Stand with proper posture.

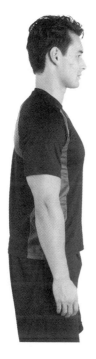

2 Pretend that you're trying to put your hands in your back pockets. Don't hold your breath. The purpose of this exercise is to teach you what it feels like to open up your chest and keep your shoulders back and down. Hold for 5–10 seconds, but don't hold so long as to cause a cramp.

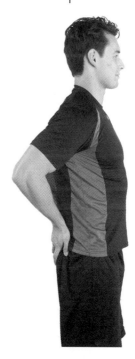

Release and relax.

Repeat as desired.

THE ZIPPER

GOAL: increase shoulder flexibility

TARGET: shoulder

You can also try this stretch while sitting or taking a warm shower.

1 Stand with proper posture. Hold a strap in one hand and raise your arm above your head, dropping the strap down your back. Bring your opposite hand up your back to grab the dangling end of the strap.

2 Raise your top hand up as high as possible to lift the lower hand, staying in your pain-free zone. Hold the position for a comfortable moment.

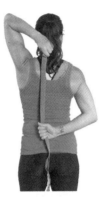

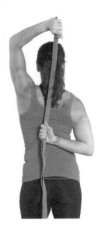

3 Now allow the lower hand to pull the higher hand down. Hold the position for a comfortable moment.

Switch sides and repeat as desired.

PROGRESSION

As you become more flexible, eliminate the use of the strap and try to grab your fingertips.

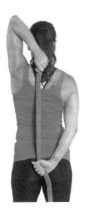

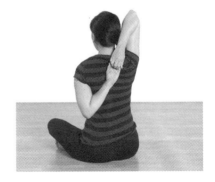

GOAL: increase strength and functional flexibility of rotator cuff muscles

TARGET: deltoids, rotator cuff

This can also be done while lying on the floor or even in bed.

1 Stand with proper posture with your affected arm at your side and elbow bent to 90 degrees. Place a rolled-up towel between your body and upper arm. Point your thumb up.

2 Keeping your elbow as close to your body as possible and your forearm parallel to the floor, rotate your forearm out to the side.

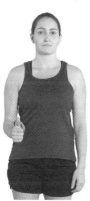

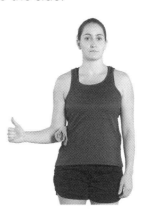

3 Rotate your forearm back in toward your body, and, if possible, place your hand on top of your belly button.

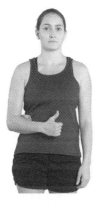

Repeat as desired and switch sides.

SUPINE VARIATION

Lie on your back with your elbows next to your body and then bend your arms 90 degrees with your elbow

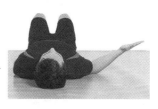

resting on the floor, fingers pointing toward the ceiling. Slowly allow the backs of your hands to lower to the floor if possible (most people won't be able to reach the floor). Don't force it; stay within a comfortable zone. Then slowly allow the palm of your hand to drop toward your belly button.

CROSSING GUARD

GOAL: increase shoulder mobility

TARGET: rotator cuff muscles

Avoid this exercise if it feels uncomfortable.

1 Lie on your back with your arms out to the sides at shoulder level. Bend your elbows 90 degrees with your hands facing forward and your fingertips pointing to the ceiling.

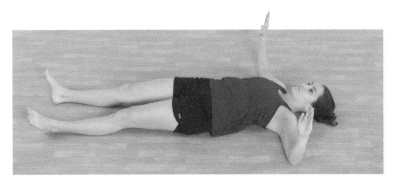

2 If possible, slowly allow the backs of your hand to drop toward the floor, staying within your comfort zone. Hold for 5–10 seconds.

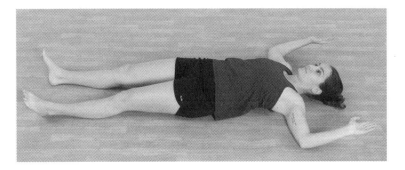

Return to start position.

Repeat as desired.

GOAL: increase external rotation of shoulder

TARGET: rotator cuff muscles

Some people find this exercise more comfortable than lying on their back.

1 Lie on your unaffected side. Rest the elbow of your affected side on your rib cage, hand in down position. You may place a towel between your torso and your elbow.

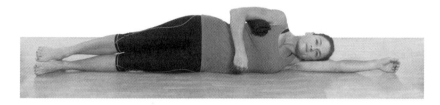

2 Slowly lift your fist up and back as high as is comfortable. Don't force the motion or do it rapidly.

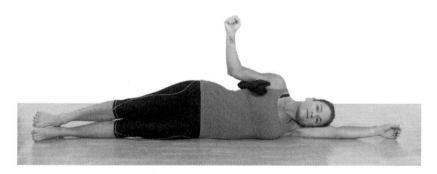

Return to start position.

Repeat as desired.

STRAIGHT-ARM STRETCH

GOAL: increase range of motion of shoulder

TARGET: shoulder girdle

1 Lying on your back, extend your affected arm toward the ceiling with your thumb pointing back. Try to keep your shoulder blades together.

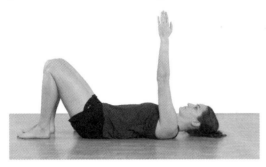

2–3 Keeping your arm straight, slowly move the arm down alongside your body, and then slowly extend the arm back toward the floor, attempting to get your thumb as close to the floor as is comfortable. Don't force the motion in either direction.

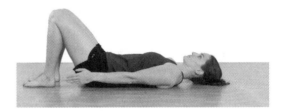

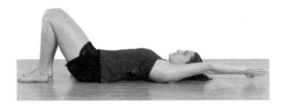

Repeat as desired, attempting to increase range each time, and then switch sides.

GOAL: increase range of motion of shoulder

TARGET: shoulder, chest

1 Lying on your back with your knees bent, raise both arms toward the ceiling.

2 Keeping your back flat, slowly move both arms directly back by your head, staying within your pain-free zone. From a top view, you'll look like an "I."

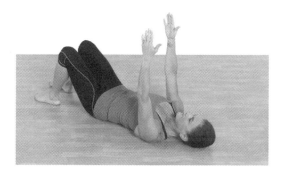

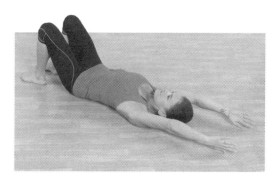

Return to start position and repeat as desired.

3 After completing the I's, take both arms back and out to the sides at a 45-degree angle to form a "Y" shape.

4 After completing the Y's, take both arms directly out to the sides to form a "T" shape.

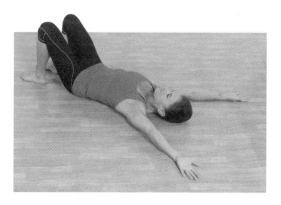

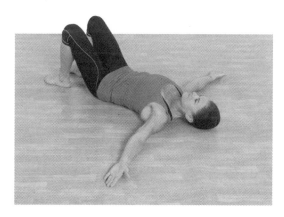

WALL PUSH-UP

GOAL: increase stabilization of shoulder girdle

TARGET: upper-back muscles

1 Stand 2 to 3 feet from a wall and place your hands shoulder-width apart on it at approximately chest height.

2 Slowly bend your elbows to lower your chest toward the wall. Focus on squeezing your shoulder blades together.

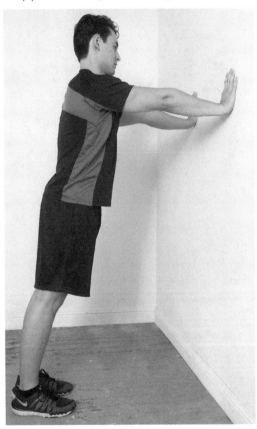

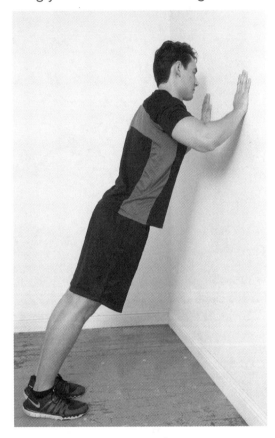

Slowly return to start position.

Repeat as desired.

GOAL: increase extension of the shoulder girdle

TARGET: shoulder blades

1 Stand with proper posture against a wall with your arms alongside your body and palms against the wall.

2 Keeping your arms straight, slowly and carefully push your palms into the wall. Hold for 3–5 seconds. Don't hold your breath or go past your safe, pain-free zone.

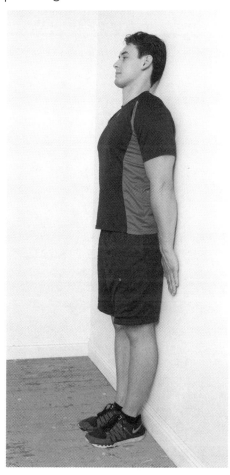

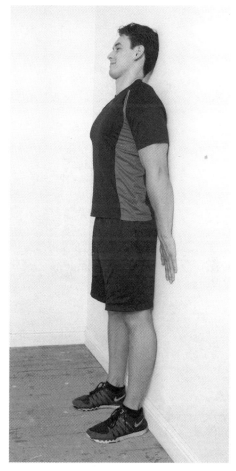

Slowly return to start position.

Repeat as desired.

THE "X"

GOAL: improve shoulder flexibility

TARGET: deltoids, rotator cuff

1 Stand with proper posture and reach the arm of your affected shoulder as high diagonally as is comfortable, keeping your palm facing forward.

2 Inhale deeply through your nose and then bring the arm down diagonally across your body toward the opposite hip. Hold for a moment.

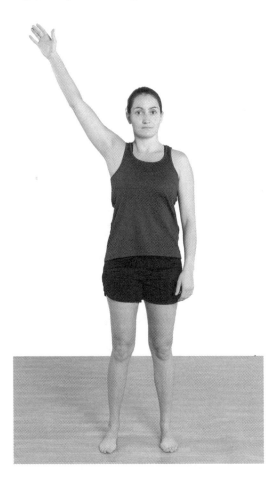
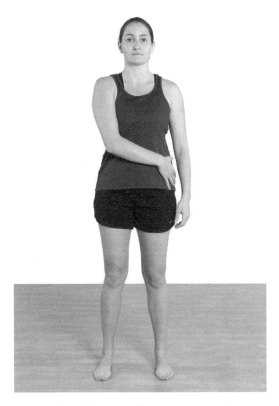

Turn your thumb up and return to start position.

Repeat as desired and switch sides.

GOAL: increase shoulder range of motion

TARGET: deltoids, upper back

If you're extremely inflexible, don't do this until you've received medical clearance.

1 Standing upright, hold a cane or stick with both hands behind your back at tailbone level.

2 Slowly move the cane or stick away from your tailbone, staying in your pain-free zone. Hold.

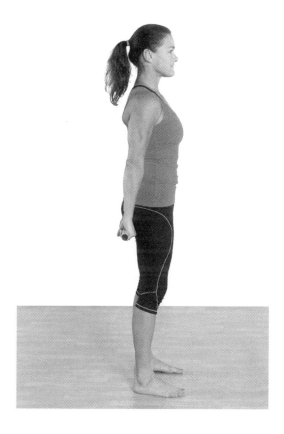
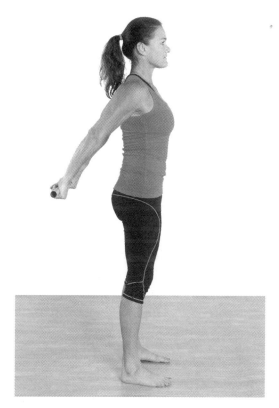

Return to start position.

Repeat as desired.

BACK RUB

GOAL: increase shoulder range of motion

TARGET: deltoids

If you're extremely inflexible, don't do this until you've received medical clearance.

1 Standing upright, hold a cane or stick with both hands behind your back at tailbone level.

2 Slowly move the cane or stick up your back, staying in your pain-free zone.

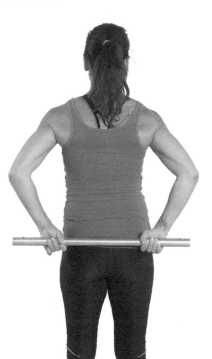

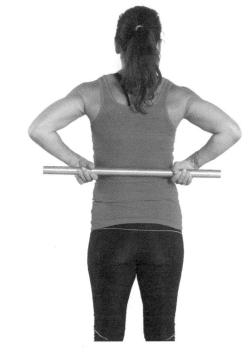

Return to start position.

Repeat as desired.

GOAL: increase chest and shoulder flexibility

TARGET: chest, shoulder

This is sometimes too uncomfortable to be done in the early stages of recovery. Use common sense to determine if you're ready.

1 Stand and place your spine along the edge/corner of a wall. Focus on keeping your lower back and head against the corner. Breathe naturally. Slowly allow your shoulder blades to wrap around the corner with the goal of opening up your chest area. Hold for 5–10 seconds.

MODIFICATION

Before performing this at the edge of a wall, try lying on a roller, allowing gravity to assist the motion.

ADVANCED VARIATION

As you improve, place your hands on your shoulders to enhance the stretch. Squeeze your shoulder blades, pulling your elbows back, and hold comfortably for 5–30 seconds. If uncomfortable, avoid and never force the motion. Release and relax. Repeat as desired.

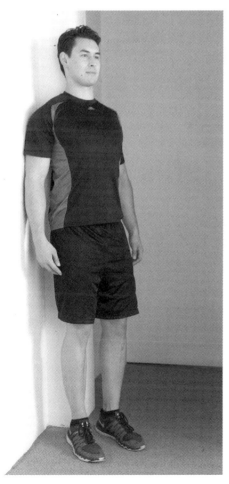

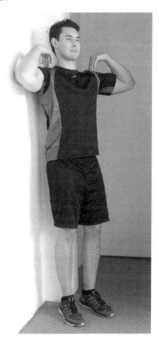

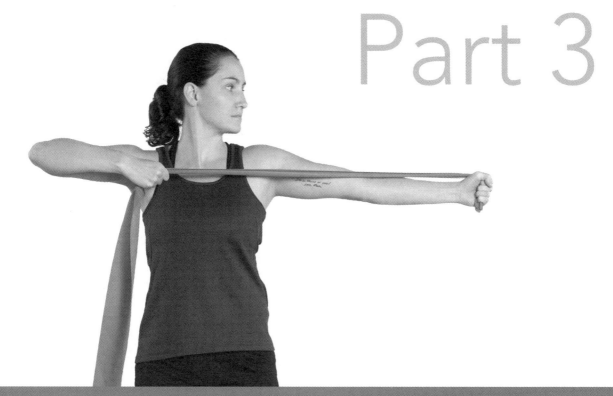

Part 3

MAINTENANCE, STRENGTHENING, & CONDITIONING EXERCISES

Chapter 6

POST-INJURY: KEEPING YOUR SHOULDER STRONG AND HEALTHY

You've worked long and hard to get past the pain of your frozen shoulder. Don't overestimate your health and re-injure yourself. If you feel ready to strengthen your weakened shoulder muscles, progress slowly as you return to more functional activities. Focus on maintaining an active range of motion. Your muscles may not have been used properly for months, so take it gently. Many frozen shoulder patients are able to redevelop their muscle power just by resuming their normal, everyday activities. However, a more focused approach may be helpful. For instance, a routine of resistance conditioning exercises is designed to improve the strength and muscle tone of the shoulder girdle.

Many people, once they fully recover, will want to return to the gym. Some people may never progress to this level, and that's fine. But for those ready to advance, keep in mind that performing advanced moves can cause a regression of symptoms if not performed correctly. Certain exercises such as lateral raises, shoulder presses, and chest exercises performed on a machine can be problematic. If you return to the gym, start far lighter than you think you can do. Remember how long it took you to recover? Returning to the gym too quickly, lifting too heavy, or doing things improperly will only re-injure you again. Consult with your health professional and use common sense when incorporating gym machines. Also, be careful of what a gym trainer tells you—many trainers are not experts in the biomechanics of exercise. When performing strength training for habilitation purposes, overstraining is *not* the goal. Your goal should be proper form and execution. When using resistance, it's important that you control the movement—don't allow the resistance to control you. Performing the movement slowly in both directions (e.g., up 2, 3 , 4, hold, down 2, 3, 4) is generally the safest bet.

Ten things to consider when designing your post-injury strength training shoulder program:

1. Build a routine that matches your interests, time restraints, and functional needs.

2. Take this book to your health professional and ask them to select some additional exercises for you to include. At this stage, you and your health provider understand your shoulder issues and should be able to design an ongoing shoulder fitness program.

3. Include exercises that offer a variety of functional movements.

4. Include periodization in your program, such as tweaking your program every six weeks by eliminating some exercises and adding new ones.

5. Only select exercises that make you feel better and that you enjoy. The best-designed program that sits in a drawer is of no use.

6. Make gains, not pain! Remember the two-hour rule: If you feel worse two hours after exercising, reevaluate the routine.

7. Stretch and flex! Every exercise routine should include a thermal warm-up, either with external heat or an active exercise to increase the blood flow and temperature of the shoulder area, followed by a few static stretches at the end of your physical activity. Consider using ice if recommended by your health professional; some therapists may suggest using kinesio tape while exercising.

8. Form = function! Poor form equates to poor body mechanics and over time insults the joint.

9. What you do to the shoulder joint today will influence you tomorrow. When performing strength training for rehabilitation purposes, avoid overstraining.

10. No pain no gain is insane! If it hurts, evaluate "why" and revise your routine.

Training Tip: As you progress to more challenging exercises, remain mindful of form and proper body mechanics. Stabilization is critical in keeping joints in biomechanical alignment.

MAINTENANCE PROGRAM

The goal of the maintenance program is to prevent any relapses. The primary focus is on general conditioning of the shoulder. This includes gentle stretching exercises as well as movements to strengthen the surrounding muscles of the shoulder complex. At this point in your recovery, you should be able to design your own program based on your skill level and needs.

POST-INJURY TIPS

If you continue doing what hurt you, expect to get hurt again. Here are some simple tips to avoid a relapse:

• Poor biomechanics or misalignments can set you up for another injury. Stay mindful that lifestyle behaviors, compounded by work duties or recreational pursuits, place additional demands on an already-compromised joint.

• As you move from injury to full recovery, consider increasing joint balance, which is the proper combination of the three S's: stretching, safety, and strength training.

• Strengthen the joint via major muscle groups, such as the deltoids.

Here are four steps to keep you on the right track.

Step 1. Warm-up exercises should include a thermal warm up of the joint region and two to three passive and active moves.

Step 2. Choose one to three functional range-of-motion exercises and two to three stretches (such as The Zipper, Cross-Shoulder Touch, and/or Finger Walking, frontal or side).

Step 3. The strengthening aspect of your program should include functional exercises that will facilitate the activities of daily lifting, such as, if possible, lifting a light weight overhead, along with exercises that address all motions of the shoulder joint (i.e., forward, side, backward).

Step 4. Lastly, a shoulder stretch session should be part of your daily routine, much like brushing your teeth. Many people combine drying off after a shower with their shoulder stretch session. It's often easier since the warm shower limbers up the shoulder joint. You can also find an isolated spot at work to stretch out your shoulder after sitting at the computer for a while or using machinery such as a jack hammer.

Fit Tip: The following routine doesn't mean you can eliminate corrective exercise nor does it supplant the daily dose of corrective exercises. The routine is only meant to supplement your corrective exercises. This is an optional program for those who desire to include strength training in their fitness routine

SAMPLE ROUTINE: Post-Injury Strength-Training Routine

Begin with a thermal warm-up and end with post-workout flexibility exercises.

Isometric External Rotation at Door, page 101

Windmill on Roller, page 103

Lat Pull-Down, page 107

Y with Band, page 113

T with Band, page 114

STRENGTH & CONDITIONING EXERCISES

The following exercises and stretches are offered as a safe and sane approach to become functionally fit. These shouldn't exacerbate your existing shoulder issues when done in a prudent manner and can be included in your total fitness program. The exercises in this section are in order of intensity, starting with isometric (static/hold) exercises and progressing to dynamic strength-training exercises with bands or weights. After the isometric exercises, the band series is where most people should begin. Resistance-band exercises should only be performed when the pain has diminished more than 90 percent and the majority of functional range of motion has returned. If discomfort returns, stop! Select only a few exercises and perform only a few reps to see how your shoulder responds. Always perform the exercises without a band first to evaluate your ability to perform the movement, then start with the easiest resistance and progress slowly. Use a high-quality resistance band product and inspect it for any damage. The way you hold the band is up to you, but try varying your grip to find the most comfortable position for the exercise. If you'd like more options on band exercises, see *Resistance Band Workbook* (Ulysses Press, 2013).

Only use dumbbells when you're on your way to 100-percent full recovery and can perform the exercise both without a weight and with a resistance band (if an option is available).

Even then, always start far lighter than you think you can do and progress from there. If you feel comfortable, try to do two sets of each exercise. As you improve, consider doing the exercises on both sides to foster symmetrical development. Progress from only doing five reps and one light set to adding weight when you can perform 10–12 reps with the weight. Since these exercises are intended for toning and conditioning, higher reps are preferred to a heavy load with lower reps. At this stage there's no reason to stop proper warm-up routines.

Caution: If pain occurs, STOP! Add and delete exercises as your shoulder suggests.

STATIC SHOULDER BLADE PUSH-UP

GOAL: stabilize shoulder blade muscle

TARGET: upper back

1 Assume a push-up position with your hands directly under your shoulders and your legs extended behind you. Your body should form a straight line from head to heels.

2 While in this position, contract your upper-back muscle to squeeze your shoulder blades together. Hold for 5–10 seconds.

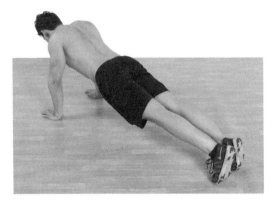

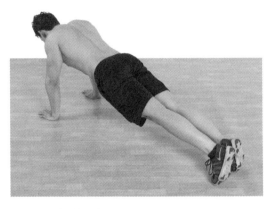

Repeat as desired.

MODIFICATION

This can also be done from your knees or with your hands against a countertop or wall.

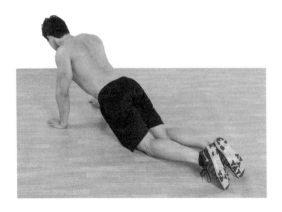

ISOMETRIC EXTERNAL ROTATION AT DOOR

GOAL: increase external rotation strength

TARGET: rotator cuff

THE POSITION: Stand sideways to a doorframe. Bend the elbow of the affected arm 90 degrees, keeping the elbow next to your ribs. Place the back of your hand against the doorframe. You may place a small pillow between your hand and the doorframe to protect your hand. Press the back of your hand into the doorframe. Hold for 3–5 seconds. Repeat as desired.

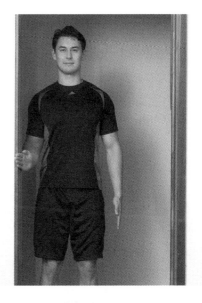

ISOMETRIC INTERNAL ROTATION AT DOOR

GOAL: increase internal rotation strength

TARGET: rotator cuff

THE POSITION: Stand facing the side of a doorframe. Bend the elbow of the affected arm 90 degrees, keeping the elbow next to your ribs. Place the palm of your hand against the doorframe. You may place a small pillow between your hand and the doorframe to protect your hand. Press your palm into the doorframe. Hold for 3–5 seconds. Repeat as desired.

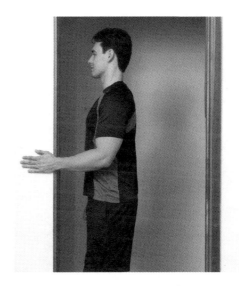

ISOMETRIC FRONTAL LIFT

GOAL: increase shoulder flexion strength

TARGET: muscle tone

THE POSITION: Stand facing a wall with the back of your hand against the wall. Push the back of your hand into the wall as if trying to lift your arm straight up. Hold for 3–5 seconds, utilizing enough tension to foster muscle tone. Repeat as desired.

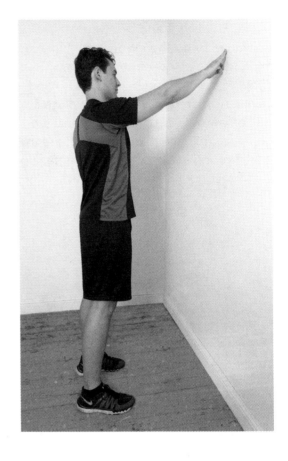

GOAL: increase range of motion and strengthen shoulder stabilization muscles

TARGET: shoulder girdle

You can also do this on the floor without a roller.

1 Lie on a foam roller from head to tail-bone with your knees bent and feet flat on floor. Allow adequate time for your upper back and shoulder region to relax onto the roller and open up. Breathe naturally and get comfortable balancing on the roller. For many people, this is an adequate enough stretch and it's okay to stop here.

2 Once comfortable and stable, extend both arms up toward the ceiling, maintaining balance on the roller.

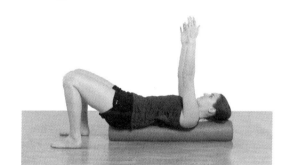

3 Tightening your core, move one arm forward and the other backward. Stay within your comfortable range of motion.

PROGRESSION

If there's no increase in pain or loss of mobility, try doing one set with your shoulder blades stabilized and one set allowing your shoulder blades to move.

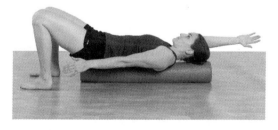

Reverse direction.

Repeat as desired.

I'S, Y'S & T'S ON ROLLER

GOAL: increase shoulder flexibility and stabilization

TARGET: chest

This is an advanced exercise. Don't do this exercise until you've completed the I's, Y's, and T's on a solid surface (page 87). You can also do this on the floor without a roller.

1 Lie on a foam roller from head to tail-bone with your knees bent and feet flat on floor. Allow adequate time for your upper back and shoulder region to relax onto the roller and open up. Breathe naturally and get comfortable balancing on the roller.

2 Once comfortable, extend both arms up toward the ceiling.

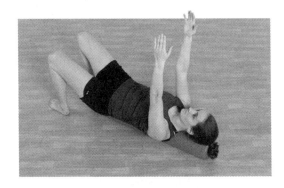

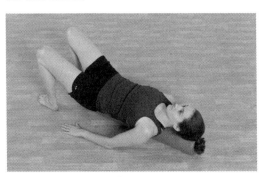

3 Now move both arms back toward the floor, making an "I" shape.

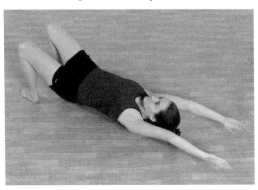

4 After completing the I's, perform the same exercise except slightly take both arms back at a 45-degree angle, forming a "Y" shape.

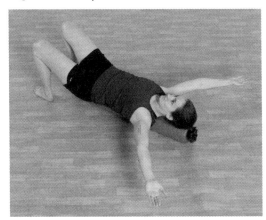

5 After completing the Y's, take both arms directly to the sides to form a "T" shape. Try to get your knuckles to the floor but don't force it.

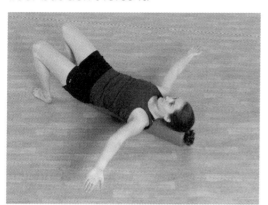

ELBOW DROP

GOAL: open chest and shoulder girdle

TARGET: chest, shoulder

You can also do this on the floor without a roller.

1 Lie on a foam roller from head to tail-bone with your knees bent and feet flat on floor. Allow adequate time for your upper back and shoulder region to relax onto the roller and open up. Breathe naturally and get comfortable balancing on the roller.

2 Once comfortable, place your palms under your head and slowly allow your elbows to "drop" toward the floor. You shouldn't expect to touch the floor. Stop if this is uncomfortable.

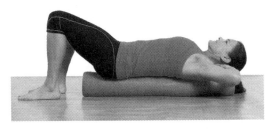

Hold the stretch while breathing naturally as tolerated.

Repeat as desired.

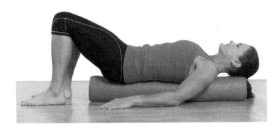

GOAL: increase shoulder and upper-back strength and scapular mobility

TARGET: lats, upper back

1 Sit in a chair with a band securely attached to the top of a door or other tall, secure object. Reach up and grab the band in each hand at a place that allows moderate resistance.

2 With arms extended, slowly pull down the band toward your chest, focusing on squeezing your shoulder blades together. As you improve and pain decreases, roll your shoulder blades forward and then pull them back when pulling the band.

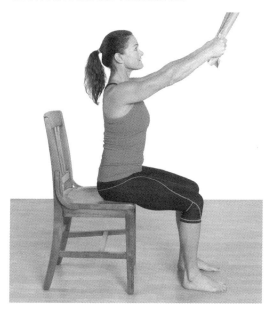

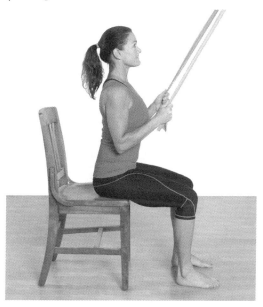

Moving only your arms and trying to keep your shoulder blades together, return to start position. Only the arms move.

Repeat as desired.

VARIATION

This exercise can be done one arm at a time.

PROGRESSION

If there's no increase in pain or loss of mobility, try doing one set with your shoulder blades stabilized and one set allowing your shoulder blades to move.

REVERSE FLY

GOAL: increase upper-back strength and scapular mobility

TARGET: upper back for posture improvement

This exercise can also be performed while sitting.

1 Stand with proper posture and grasp the band in each hand. Extend your arms in front of your shoulders, keeping your arms parallel to the floor, your wrists neutral (don't bend them), and your head and upper back in proper alignment.

2 Inhale and slowly open your arms out to the sides while keeping your arms straight and parallel to the floor.

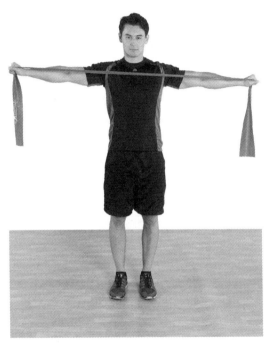

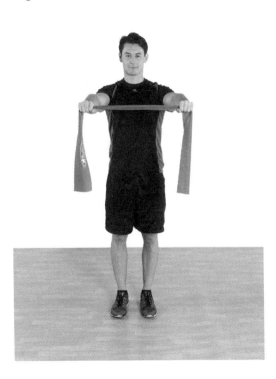

Return to start position. Repeat as desired.

GOAL: improve posture

TARGET: biceps, upper back

This exercise can also be performed while sitting.

1 Stand with proper posture. Hold one end of a band in your left hand and extend your left arm straight out to the side. With your right hand, grasp the band near your left elbow or shoulder at a location that provides proper resistance.

2 Pull your right arm across your chest, drawing your elbow to your right side.

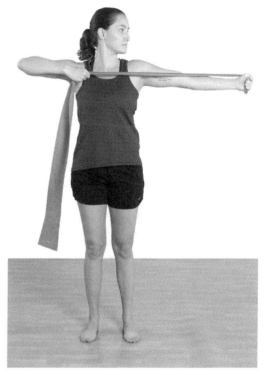

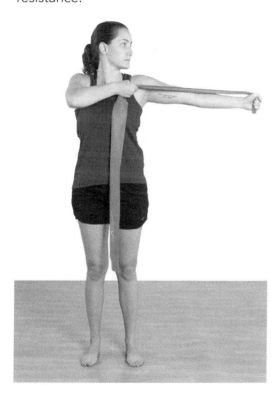

Slowly return to start position.

Repeat as desired, and then switch sides.

CHEST PRESS

GOAL: stabilize shoulder

TARGET: chest, anterior shoulder

This exercise can also be performed while sitting.

1 Stand with proper posture and place a band around your back at chest height. Grasp the band with each hand at a place that provides moderate resistance.

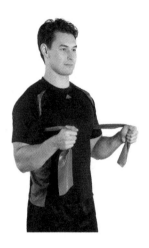

2 While focusing on keeping your shoulder blades back and stable, press your arms forward.

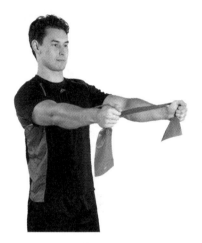

Control the motion as the arms return to start position. Don't allow the band to recoil you.

Repeat as desired.

VARIATION

This can also be performed with one arm at a time.

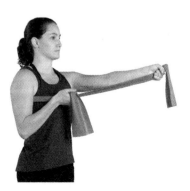

PROGRESSION

If there's no increase in pain or loss of mobility, try doing one set with your shoulder blades stabilized and one set allowing your shoulder blades to move.

GOAL: improve shoulder stabilization

TARGET: deltoid muscles

This advanced exercise can also be performed while sitting. Be careful.

1 Stand with proper posture and place a band around your back and under your armpits. Grasp the band in each hand at a place that provides moderate resistance.

2 Keeping your shoulder blades together, press your arms upward until they're fully extended. The amount of upward motion is dependent upon your flexibility and pain tolerance. Some people can't go directly up, and that's okay. Your focus should be on replicating the functional motions of putting something in an overhead luggage bin, so a slight angle is fine.

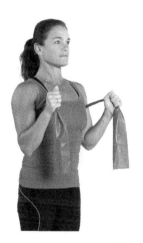

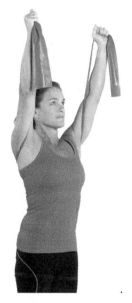

PROGRESSION

If there's no increase in pain or loss of mobility, try doing one set with your shoulder blades stabilized and one set allowing your shoulder blades to move.

Control the motion as the arms return to start position. Don't let the band recoil you.

Repeat as desired.

GRADUATED PRESS

GOAL: improve functional mobility

TARGET: chest muscles

A blend of a horizontal chest press, incline chest press, and shoulder press, this exercise can also be performed while sitting.

1 Stand with proper posture and place a band around your mid-upper back. Grasp the band with each hand at a place that provides moderate resistance.

2 Keeping your wrists neutral (don't bend them) and your head and upper back in proper posture, slowly press both ends of the band forward. Pause when your arms are extended in front of you then slowly return to start position. Repeat 3–5 times.

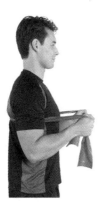

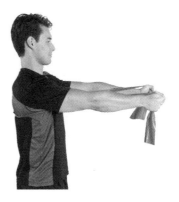

3 Perform another 3–5 reps, this time slowly pressing both ends of the band forward and upward at a 45-degree angle.

4 If comfortable, perform another 3–5 reps, pressing both ends of the band directly upward toward the ceiling.

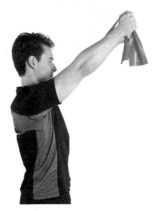

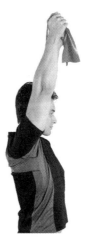

GOAL: increase shoulder girdle muscle strength and mobility

TARGET: upper back and rear deltoid muscles

This exercise can also be performed while sitting.

1 Stand with proper posture. Grasp the band with your hands shoulder-width apart and raise your arms overhead as high as is comfortable.

2 Keeping your head straight and shoulder blades squeezed together, slowly pull the band apart to the sides until your hands are about shoulder level.

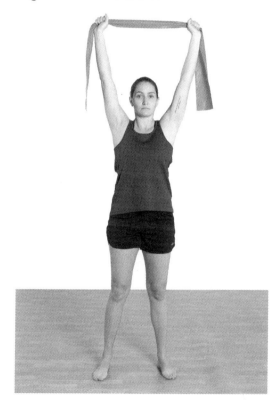

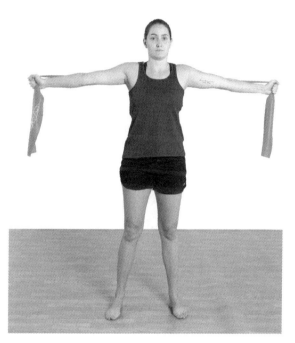

Slowly return to start position.

Repeat as desired.

T WITH BAND

GOAL: strengthen muscles behind the shoulder blades, improve posture, and provide scapular stabilization

TARGET: scapula

1 Stand with proper posture and grasp the band with your hands shoulder-width apart, palms down. Don't wrap the band around your hands. Keeping your arms straight, raise your hands to approximately shoulder height.

2 Squeezing the muscles that bring your should blades together, slowly open your arms out to the sides.

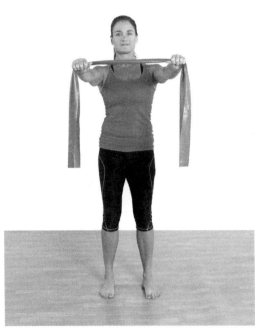

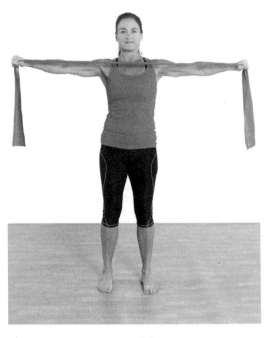

Slowly return to start position.

Repeat as desired.

GOAL: increase shoulder flexion strength

TARGET: deltoids

Approach this exercise with caution as some people find this move uncomfortable.

1 Standing with proper posture, place one end of a band under one foot and grasp the other end with one hand, thumb facing up. Avoid performing this with your palm facing down or up as this could be harmful. Adjust resistance by moving your hand up or down the band. Resistance should be felt when you start raising your arm. Arm should be straight as possible but not locked.

2 Keeping your arm straight, slowly bring your arm up to shoulder height. If this is comfortable, raise your arm all the way up. If this is at all uncomfortable, lower your arm to start position.

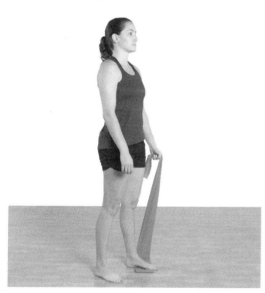

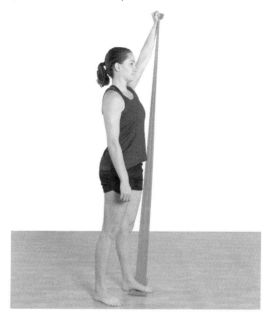

Repeat and then switch sides.

DUMBBELL VARIATION

Instead of a band, hold a dumbbell with your palm facing your thigh or your thumb up. Slowly lift your arm forward no 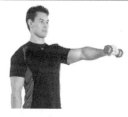 higher than shoulder level, staying within your pain-free range of motion.

LATERAL ARM RAISE

GOAL: increase abduction strength of shoulder

TARGET: medial portion of the deltoid

Approach this exercise with caution as some people find this move uncomfortable.

1 Standing with proper posture, place one end of a band under the foot of your affected side and grasp the band with the same-side hand, palm down or thumb up.

2 Slowly raise your arm to the side to shoulder height. If this is uncomfortable, move your arm to a different angle to find a "comfort" zone. If this is still uncomfortable, don't do this movement.

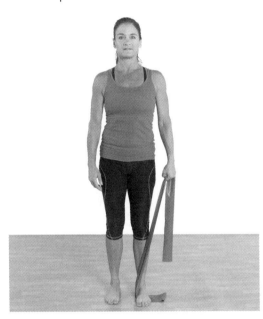

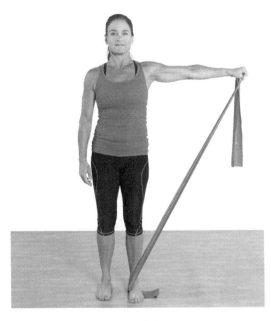

Slowly return to start position.

Repeat and then switch sides.

VARIATION

This can also be done with dumbbells.

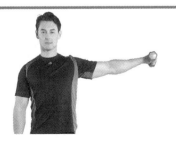

GOAL: increase shoulder extension strength

TARGET: anterior deltoid

Stay mindful of your safe range of motion.

1 Standing with proper posture, place one end of a band under the foot of your affected side and grasp the band with the same-side hand, thumb up. Stay within your pain-free zone.

2 Keeping your arm straight, slowly move the arm backward.

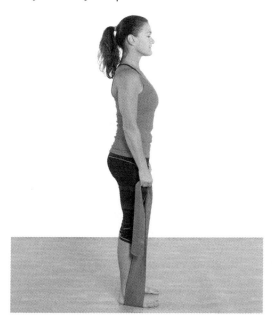

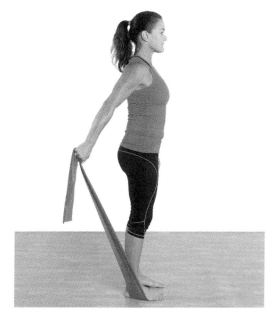

Return to start position.

VARIATION

This can also be done with dumbbells.

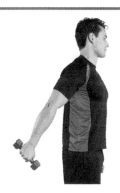

SWORD FIGHTER

GOAL: increase upper-shoulder and back strength

TARGET: posterior deltoid

1 Standing with proper posture, place the arm of your unaffected side alongside your body and hold on to a band. With the hand of the affected shoulder, grasp the other end of the band at a place that provides mild resistance.

2 Pull the hand of the affected shoulder diagonally across your body as if pulling a sword out of its sheath.

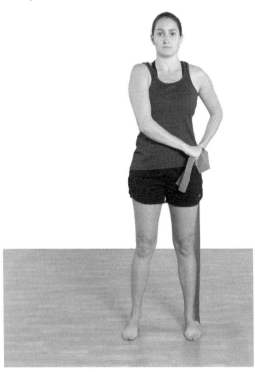

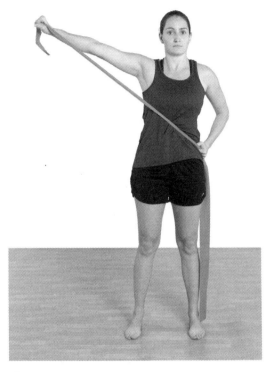

Slowly return to start position.

Repeat.

GOAL: increase rotator cuff strength

TARGET: rotator cuff

1 Standing with proper posture, bend both elbows 90 degrees and place a band across elbows next to your ribs. Now grasp the band with both palms up, keeping both wrists neutral to avoid any wrist pain.

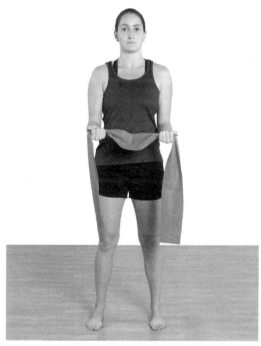

2 Slowly move your hands away from each other as if serving appetizers. Hold for 3–5 seconds.

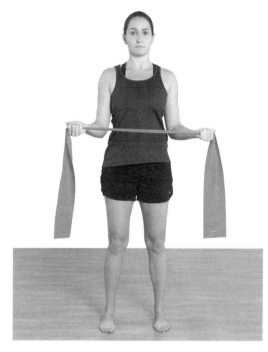

Return to start position and repeat.

MODIFICATION

If this feels uncomfortable, try one arm at a time (keep one hand in place while the other moves to the outside, or tie one end securely to a doorknob) or perform the Isometric External Rotation at Door (page 101).

SINGLE-ARM INTERNAL ROTATION

GOAL: increase internal rotation strength

TARGET: rotator cuff

1 Attach the end of an exercise band securely to a doorknob or another solid object and position your affected side closest to the doorknob. Be care that it doesn't come loose. Grasp the band, bend your elbow 90 degrees, and place your elbow next to your ribs. Keep your wrist neutral to avoid any wrist pain. You may place a rolled-up towel or small pillow between your elbow and your body.

2 Slowly move your hand across your body as if to place your palm over your belly button.

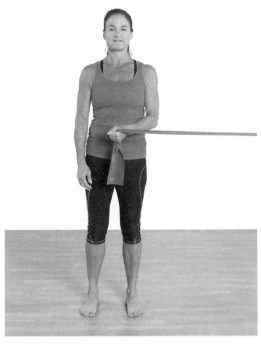

Slowly return to start position.

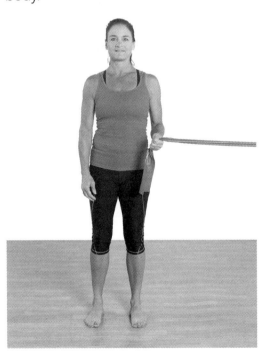

MODIFICATION

If this feels uncomfortable, perform the Isometric Internal Rotation at Door (page 101).

GOAL: increase external rotation strength

TARGET: rotator cuff

1 Attach the end of an exercise band securely to a doorknob or another solid object and position your affected side away from the doorknob. Be careful that it doesn't come loose. Grasp the band, place your elbow next to your ribs; hand position is in front of hip. Keep your wrist neutral to avoid any wrist pain. You may place a rolled-up towel or small pillow between your elbow and your body.

2 Slowly move your hand away from the doorknob.

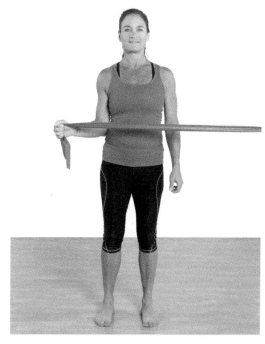

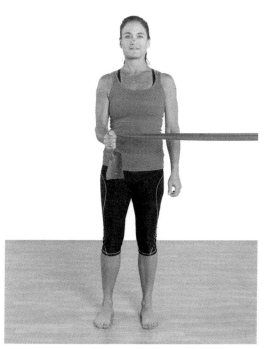

Slowly return to start position.

SEATED ROW WITH BAND

GOAL: increase upper-back strength

TARGET: upper back

1 Place a band around the foot on your affected side, grasp the band with both hands at a place that provides adequate resistance, and extend your leg in front of you.

2 Slowly pull the band toward your torso, pulling your shoulder blades together.

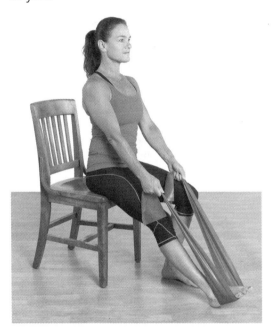

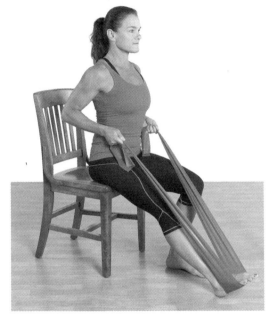

Slowly return to start position.

OPTION AS YOU IMPROVE

See how it feels if you allow your shoulders blades to glide as you perform this exercise. If there is no increase in pain or loss of mobility, try doing one set with shoulder blades stabilized and one set allowing shoulder blades to move.

GOAL: increase upper-back strength and shoulder stabilization

TARGET: shoulder

This version is more advanced than the band version on page 108.

1 Lie facedown on a bench with your chin resting on the bench. Hold a dumbbell in the hand of your affected arm and let it hang off the side of the bench.

2 Slowly raise your arm to a parallel position with the floor.

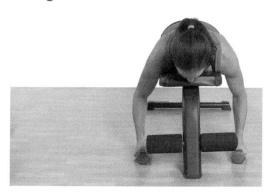

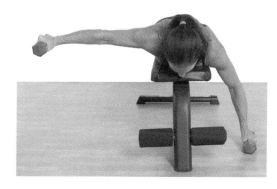

Slowly return to start position. Repeat as desired.

SOUP CAN POUR WITH WEIGHT

GOAL: increase shoulder girdle stabilization and functional mobility

TARGET: deltoids, rotator cuff

1 Standing with proper posture, hold a dumbbell in the hand of your affected arm. Turn your thumb down with palm facing backward.

2 Staying mindful of keeping your thumb down and moving within your pain-free zone, slowly lift your arm out to the side at a 45-degree angle.

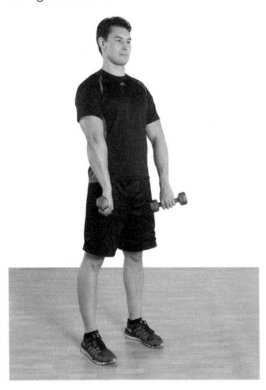

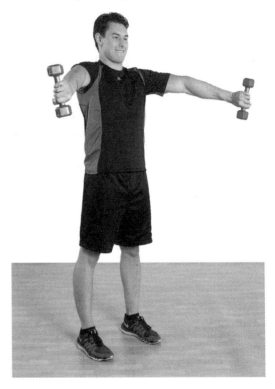

Lower slowly.

GOAL: increase shoulder girdle strength

TARGET: trapezius

1 Standing with proper posture, hold a dumbbell in each hand.

2 Inhaling slowly and deeply through your nose, shrug your shoulders up.

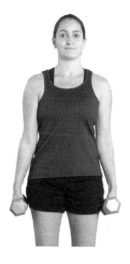

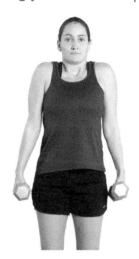

3 Exhaling though your lips, squeeze your shoulder blades together as you slowly lower them back down to start position.

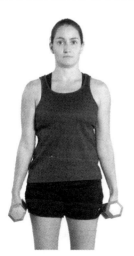

At the completion of the exercise, you have outlined the shape of a box.

HANGING DUMBBELL SQUEEZE

GOAL: increase upper-body strength, traction, and stabilization

TARGET: rhomboids

1 Bend over a sturdy table or chair while supporting yourself with your unaffected arm; bend your knees to prevent strain on your lower back. Grab a light dumbbell with your affected arm and allow the dumbbell to pull gently down on your arm.

2 Squeeze your shoulder blade up and together. You won't have much movement in the arm—this is a subtle motion of the shoulder blade only. Hold for 3–5 seconds.

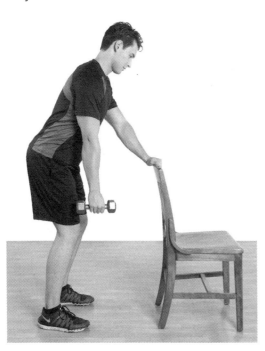

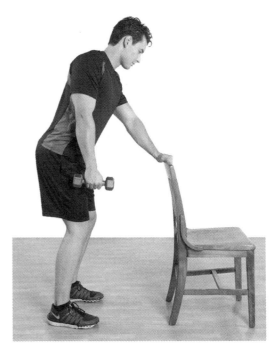

Slowly release and lower.

GOAL: increase upper-body strength, traction, and stabilization

TARGET: rhomboids, lats

1 Bend over a sturdy table or chair while supporting yourself with your unaffected arm; bend your knees to prevent strain in your lower back. Grab a medium dumbbell with your affected arm and allow the dumbbell to pull gently down on your arm.

2 Squeeze your shoulder blade up and together while you lift the weight toward your armpit.

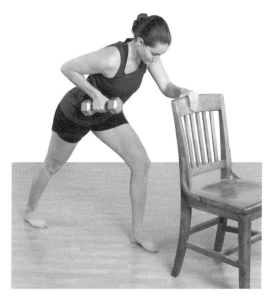

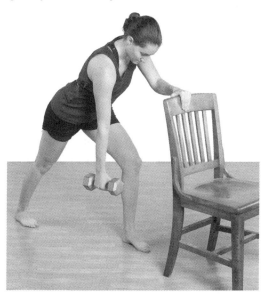

Slowly release and lower. Repeat.

WATER EXERCISES

Water exercise is an excellent therapeutic modality. One advantage is that it provides resistance in all directions and it's difficult to apply too much load. As your condition and strength improve, try increasing the resistance by using cupped hands, aqua gloves, or hand paddles. When doing water exercises you can either count reps or perform for a specific amount of time, such as 30 seconds to 1 minute. Another beauty of water exercise is that you can combine aerobic conditioning, such as jogging in place or performing jumping jacks, while performing flexibility training and muscle conditioning all in one session. For more details on water exercise, see *Make the Pool Your Gym* (Ulysses Press, 2012).

The following are some samples done standing up in the pool.

ELBOW TOUCH

GOAL: improve flexibility of chest and upper-back region

TARGET: pec muscle, rhomboid muscle

1 Stand tall with proper posture and place your right hand on your right shoulder and your left hand on your left shoulder.

2 Keeping your hands in place, slowly bring your elbows together as far as is comfortable. Hold for 5–15 seconds. Focus on squeezing your shoulder blades together and opening up your chest.

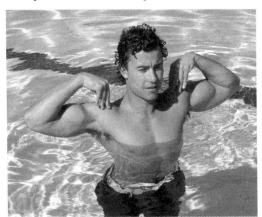

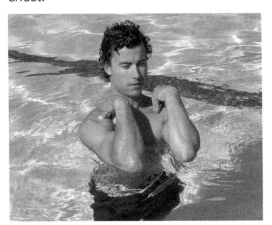

Repeat.

GOAL: functional mobility of arms and shoulder complex

TARGET: biceps, triceps, trapezius, shoulders

1–2 Hold your hands near your armpits. Press your right arm down. As you bring your right arm up, simultaneously press your left arm down.

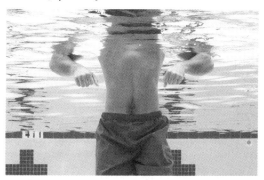 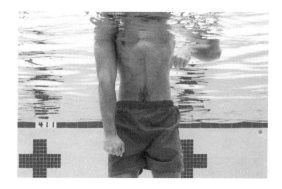

JUMPING JACK ARMS (SIDE)

GOAL: functional muscular conditioning of arms and shoulder area in the lateral direction

TARGET: shoulders (lateral)

1–2 Keeping your arms straight, quickly lift your arms sideways to the surface of the water. Keep your arms underwater—you get the resistance from the water, not the air.

Quickly return to starting position and repeat.

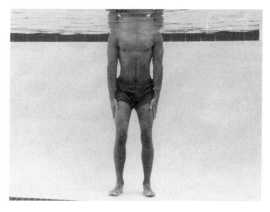 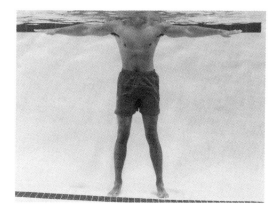

JUMPING JACK ARMS (FRONTAL)

GOAL: functional muscular conditioning of arms and shoulder area in the frontal direction

TARGET: shoulders (frontal)

1–2 Rest your arms along your sides. Keeping your arms straight, quickly lift them forward to the surface of the water. Keep your arms under-water—you get the resistance from the water, not the air.

Quickly return to starting position and repeat.

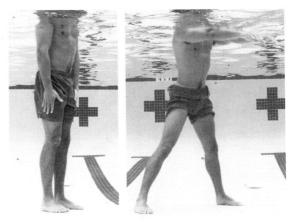

WOOD CHOP IN POOL

GOAL: improvement of overhead range of motion

TARGET: anterior deltoid muscles/shoulders

1 Stand tall with proper neutral posture. Interlace your fingers in front of your body.

2 Inhale deeply through your nose while slowly lifting your arms as high as possible. Hold for 5–10 seconds.

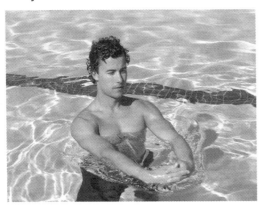

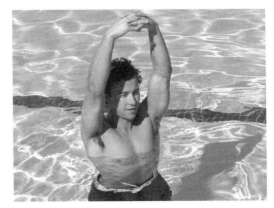

Slowly lower your arms to starting position.

POST-RECOVERY STRETCHES

Post-rehab warm-up is recommended. Make sure to take a few minutes to perform a few of these movements before and after exercise. For more detailed information on stretching, see *Stretching for 50+* (Ulysses Press, 2017).

HEAD TILT

TARGET: neck

You can also perform this active stretch while sitting.

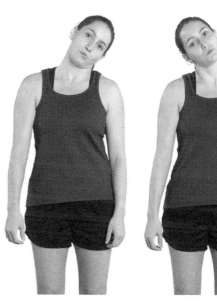

1 Stand with proper posture. While inhaling slowly through your nose, slowly tilt your head toward your left shoulder. Keep your shoulders down and relaxed. Exhale slowly through your lips and hold this position for a moment, feeling the stretch.

2 Now inhale slowly through your nose and slowly tilt your head to your right shoulder. Exhale slowly through your lips and hold this position for a moment, feeling the stretch.

WOOD CHOP

TARGET: deltoids

This is an active stretch.

1 Stand with proper posture. Position your hands in front of your body and interlace your fingers.

2 Inhale deeply through your nose and slowly raise both arms in front of you to a comfortable height. Hold for 1–2 seconds.

Slowly lower your arms to start position.

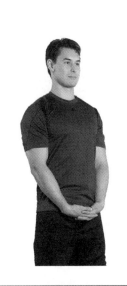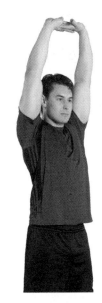

APPLE PICKER

TARGET: deltoids

This is an active stretch.

1 Stand with proper posture and place your hands on your shoulders. Reach your right hand as high as is comfortable.

2 Place your right hand back on your shoulder. Now reach up with your left hand.

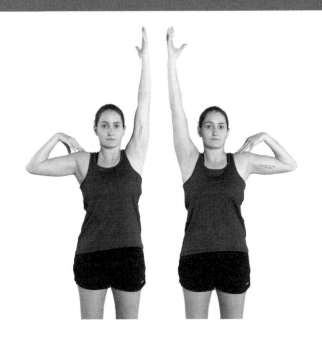

TARGET: deltoids, rotator cuff

You can also perform this active stretch while sitting.

1 Stand with proper posture with your arms at your sides and your palms facing back.

2 Inhale deeply through your nose and bring both arms slightly forward as you raise them out to the sides no higher than shoulder level, keeping your palms facing back.

Exhale as you lower your arms.

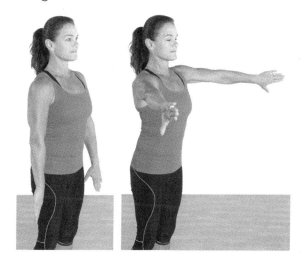

ROTATOR CUFF STRETCH

TARGET: deltoids, rotator cuff

You can also perform this active stretch while sitting.

1 Stand with proper posture, bend your right elbow 90 degrees, and point your thumb up. Squeeze a towel between your right arm and your torso.

2 Keeping your elbow as close to your body as possible and your forearm parallel to the floor, rotate your forearm out to the side.

Rotate your forearm back in toward your body.

Repeat, and then switch sides.

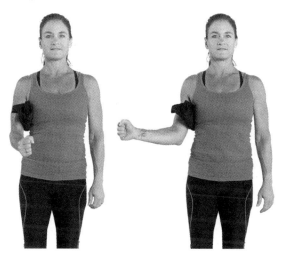

ELBOW TOUCH (STANDING)

TARGET: chest, shoulder retractor

You can also perform this active stretch while sitting.

1 Stand with proper posture and place your hands on your shoulders. Slowly bring your elbows together in front of your body.

2 Take your elbows back while squeezing your shoulder blades together. Hold for a moment, focusing on opening up your chest. Return to start position.

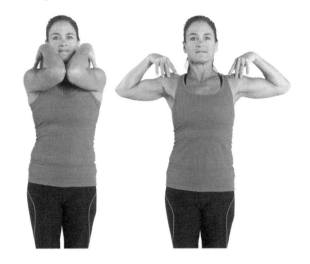

SHOULDER ROLL

TARGET: trapezius

You can also perform this static stretch while sitting.

1 Stand with proper posture. Inhale slowly and deeply through your nose. Exhaling through your nose, roll your shoulders forward, attempting to spread your shoulder blades apart.

2 Inhale and move your shoulders back, focusing on squeezing your shoulder blades together and opening up your chest. Hold for 2 counts.

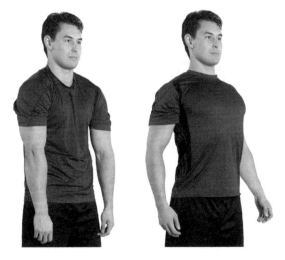

TARGET: shoulders, rotator cuff

You can also perform this static stretch while sitting.

1 Stand with proper posture and place your right hand on your left shoulder.

2 Place your left hand on your right elbow and gently press your right elbow toward your throat. Hold for a comfortable moment.

Switch sides.

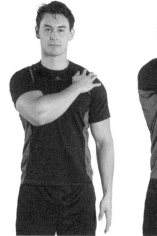
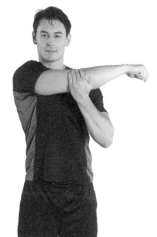

TARGET: shoulders

You can also perform this static stretch while sitting.

1 Stand with proper posture. Place your right hand on your left elbow and your left hand on your right elbow.

2 Slowly raise your arms overhead, lifting your arms as high as feels comfortable. Don't arch your lower back. Hold for a moment. You're now framing your face in a picture frame created by your arms—smile.

Switch sides, with the other hand on top.

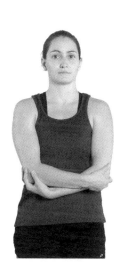
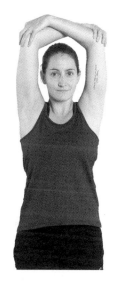

INDEX

ACKNOWLEDGMENTS

A special thanks goes out to Casie Vogel for her vision, along with the behind-the-scenes team at Ulysses Press. A special shout out goes to Lily Chou and Claire Chun, as well as the rest of the editorial team, for making sense of my writing.

Another thought of appreciation goes to the photographer Anja Ulfeldt of Rapt Productions and models Evan Clontz, Kym Sterner, and Chris Wells.

Thank you to my son Chris for his critical suggestions on content and serving as a model in the water exercise poses, and my wife Margaret for her patience. And let's not leave out my other son Kevin for reminding me to laugh.

ABOUT THE AUTHOR

Dr. Karl Knopf (or Dr. Karl, as his students called him) was the director of the fitness therapy program at Foothill College for almost 40 years. During his tenure, he received several awards for teaching excellence. He retired in 2013. During his 45-plus years in the health and fitness industry, he has worked in almost every aspect of the industry, including personal trainer (before the term was named), therapist at a VA hospital, and advisor to the State of California as well as to several National Institutes of Health grants. During his career he was a frequent speaker at national conferences and regional hospitals, and has appeared on public television's *Sit and Be Fit* show as well as a regular guest on radio.

Over the years Dr. Knopf has been interviewed for many print media publications, including the *Los Angeles Times* and *San Jose Mercury News*, and was featured in the *Wall Street Journal* on issues pertaining to senior fitness, exercise, and the disabled. He still authors articles and is still sought after for interviews. His Ulysses Press books (*Make the Pool Your Gym*, *Stretching for 50+*, *Weights for 50+*, and *Core Strength for 50+)* are promoted in Tufts University health newsletters.

Currently, Dr. Knopf is the director of fitness therapy and senior fitness for the International Sports Science Association (ISSA) and is on the executive board of *Sit and Be Fit*. Dr. Knopf walks the talk as a person who's over 65 years old. He still lifts weights, bikes, and swims daily while living with a chronic back condition for over 30-plus years. Dr. Karl understands firsthand the benefits of daily corrective exercise and firmly believes that what you do today determines if you'll be healthy and functional tomorrow. His motto is "Grow well!"